Sajeesh Kumar   Elizabeth A. Krupinski   (Eds.)

Teleradiology

Sajeesh Kumar   Elizabeth A. Krupinski (Eds.)

Teleradiology

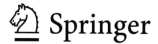 Springer

Sajeesh Kumar, Ph.D.
Department of Health Information Management
School of Health & Rehabilitation Sciences
University of Pittsburgh
6051 Forbes Tower
Pittsburgh, PA 15260
sajeeshkr@yahoo.com

Elizabeth A. Krupinski, Ph.D.
Department of Radiology
University of Arizona
1609 N. Warren Bldg 211
Tucson, AZ 85724, USA
krupinski@radiology.arizona.edu

ISBN 978-3-540-78870-6   e-ISBN 978-3-540-78871-3
DOI: 10.1007/978-3-540-78871-3

Library of Congress Catalog Number: 2008924362

Cover design: WMX Design GmbH, Heidelberg

Printed on acid-free paper

9 8 7 6 5 4 3 2 1

springer.com

Preface

Developments in teleradiology are progressing at great speed. As a consequence, there is a need for a broad overview of the field. This first-ever book on teleradiology is presented in such a way that it should make it accessible to anyone, independent of their knowledge of technology. The text is designed to be used by *all* professionals, including radiologists, surgeons, nurses and allied health professionals, and computer scientists.

In a very short time, driven by technical developments, the field of teleradiology has become too extensive to be covered by only a small number of experts. Therefore, *Teleradiology* has been written with chapter contributions from a host of renowned international authorities in teleradiology (see the Contents and the Contributors). This ensures that the subject matter focusing on recent advances in teleradiology is truly up to date. Our guiding hope during this task was that as editors of multiple chapters we could still write with a single voice and keep the content coherent and simple. We hope that the clarity of this book makes up for any limitations in its comprehensiveness.

The editors took much care so that *Teleradiology* would not become merely a collection of separate chapters but, rather, would offer a consistent and structured overview of the field. We are aware that there is still considerable room for improvement and that certain elements of teleradiology are not fully covered, such as legal matters and reimbursement policy. The editors invite readers, clinicians, and students to forward their valuable comments and feedback to further improve and expand future editions of *Teleradiology*.

Books on theoretical and technical aspects inevitably use technical jargon, and this book is no exception. Although use of jargon has been minimized, it cannot be eliminated without retreating to a more superficial level of coverage. The reader's understanding of the jargon will vary depending on his or her background, but anyone with some background in computers, health, and/or biomedicine would be able to understand most of the terms used. In any case, an attempt to define all jargon terms has been made in the Glossary.

Teleradiology has been organized systematically. The format and length of each chapter are standardized, thus ensuring that the content is concise and easy to read. Every chapter provides a comprehensive list of citations and references for further reading. Numerous drawings and clinical photographs throughout the book illustrate and illuminate the text well, providing its readers with high-quality visual reference material. Particularly useful features of this text are that each chapter has a summary of salient points for the reader.

The book comprises 21 chapters and begins with a brief introductory chapter explaining the basic concepts that are the mainstay of teleradiology, and subsequent chapters are built on those foundations. Within each chapter, the goal is to provide a comprehensive overview of the topic. The chapters on telemedicine law are deliberately placed in this first edition of the book to emphasize the fundamental importance of these topics. Nevertheless, its content is not inclusive, since opportunities are progressively arising in this domain. The final chapter covers future directions of teleradiology.

This book would not have been possible without the contribution of various people. We acknowledge and appreciate the assistance of all reviewers and Latika Hans, editorial assistant from Bangalore, India. We would like to thank all authors for making this book possible through their contributions and constant support.

SAJEESH KUMAR and ELIZABETH A. KRUPINSKI

Contents

Chapter 4
**DICOM Image Secure Communication with
Internet Protocols**............................... **33**
JIANGUO ZHANG

Chapter 5
Radiological Tele-immersion........................ **49**
ZHUMING AI, BEI JIN, and MARY RASMUSSEN

Chapter 6
**Use of a Radiology Picture Archiving and Communication
System to Catalogue Photographic Images 65**
JAMES E. SILBERZWEIG and AZITA S. KHORSANDI

Chapter 7
Teleradiology with DICOM E-mail 71
PETER MILDENBERGER

List of Contributors

B. J. J. Abdullah
Department of Biomedical Imaging
Faculty of Medicine
University of Malaya
Kuala Lumpur
Malaysia

Zhuming Ai
3D Virtual and Mixed Environments (Code 5580)
Naval Research Laboratory
4555 Overlook Ave. SW
Washington, DC 20375
USA

Ricanthony Ashley
Radiology Department
Landstuhl Regional Medical Center
CMR 402
APO AE 09180
USA

Pantelis A. Asvestas
Institute of Communication and Computer Systems
9 Iroon Polytechneiou st., Zografos
157 80 Athens
Greece

Michael Blaivas
Professor of Emergency Medicine
Northside Hospital Forsyth
Atlanta, Georgia
USA

Edward C. Callaway
Berghaldenstrasse 52b
8053 Zurich
Switzerland

Christian Compagnone
Intensive Care Unit
M. Bufalini Hospital
47023 Cesena
Italy

Fabien Courreges
Laboratoire Xlim
Dpt. Math. Info, projet CANSO
Université de Limoges
Institut Universitaire de Technologie du
Limousin Dpt. Génie Mécanique et Productique
Allée Andrée Maurois
87100 Limoges Cedex
France

Kostantinos K. Delibasis
Institute of Communication and Computer Systems
9 Iroon Polytechneiou st., Zografos
157 80 Athens
Greece

Rolf Ewers
Medical University of Vienna
University Hospital of Cranio-Maxillofacial and Oral Surgery
Waehringer Guertel 18–20
1090 Vienna
Austria

Lefteris G. Gortzis
Medical Physics Department
University of Patras
265 00 Patras
Greece

Bradley C. Heraly
Evanston Northwestern Hospital
1000 Central St, Suite 720
Evanston, IL 60201
USA

Corrado Iaccarino
Neurosurgical Unit "Hub & Spoke"
PARMA-REGGIO EMILIA
Emergency Department
University Hospital of Parma
Viale Gramsci 14, 43100 Parma
Italy

Bei Jin
Virtual Reality in Medicine Lab
Department of Biomedical and Health Information Sciences
College of Applied Health Sciences
University of Illinois at Chicago
1919 W. Taylor St., AHP, MC 530
Chicago, IL 60612
USA

William K. Johnston III
Feinberg School of Medicine
Northwestern University
Chicago, IL
USA
and
Laparoscopy and Minimally Invasive Urology
Evanston Northwestern Hospital
1000 Central St, Suite 720
Evanston, IL 60201
USA

Vassilios Kouloulias
Radiotherapy Unit
2nd Department of Radiology
Medical School
Attikon University Hospital
University of Athens, Athens
Greece

Azita S. Khorsandi
Department of Radiology
Beth Israel Medical Center
First Avenue at 16th Street
New York, NY 10003
USA

Sajeesh Kumar
Centre of Excellence in e-Medicine
University of Western Australia
2 Verdun Street, Nedlands, WA 6009
Australia

Elizabeth A. Krupinski
Department of Radiology
University of Arizona
1609 N. Warren Bldg 211
Tucson, AZ 85724
USA

David M. Lam
US Army Telemedicine and Advanced Technology Research Center
504 Scott Street
Ft. Detrick, MD 21702
USA
and
University of Maryland Medical School
(National Study Center for Trauma and EMS)
Baltimore, MD
USA

Rajasvaran Logeswaran
Centre for Image Processing and Telemedicine
Multimedia University
63100 Cyberjaya
Malaysia

George K. Matsopoulos
Department of Electrical and Computer Engineering
National Technical University of Athens
9 Iroon Polytechneiou st., Zografos
157 80 Athens
Greece

Patrick B. McLean
Third Millennium Consultants and
Eastern Kansas VA Health Care System
USA

Thomas R. McLean
4970 Park
Shawnee, KS 66216
USA

Kenneth Meade
212th Combat Support Hospital
Box 684, LRMC CMR 402
APO AE 09180
USA

Nikolaos A. Mouravliansky
Institute of Communication and Computer Systems
9 Iroon Polytechneiou st., Zografos
157 80 Athens
Greece

Peter Mildenberger
Universitätsklinikum Mainz
Langenbeckstr. 1
55131 Mainz
Germany

Ivan Ng
Department of Neurosurgery
National Neuroscience Institute, Singapore
11 Jalan Tan Tock Seng
Singapore 308433
Singapore

Wai Hoe Ng
Department of Neurosurgery
National Neuroscience Institute, Singapore
11 Jalan Tan Tock Seng
Singapore 308433
Singapore

Gérard Poisson
Laboratoire Vision & Robotique
Université d'Orléans
IUT de Bourges
63 avenue de Lattre de Tassigny
18020 Bourges Cedex
France

Ayis T. Pyrros
Northwestern Memorial Hospital
676 North St. Clair Street, Suite 800
Chicago, IL 60611-2927
USA

Ronald Poropatich
US Army Telemedicine and Advanced Technology Research Center
504 Scott Street
Ft. Detrick, MD 21702
USA

Armando Rapana'
Neurosurgical Unit
Department of Neurological Sciences
A.O.R.N. "San Sebastiano & San Anna"
Via Palasciano, 81100 Caserta
Italy

Mary Rasmussen
Virtual Reality in Medicine Lab
Department of Biomedical and Health Information Sciences
College of Applied Health Sciences
University of Illinois at Chicago
1919 W. Taylor St., AHP, MC 530
Chicago, IL 60612
USA

Jarmo Reponen
FinnTelemedicum
Centre of Excellence for Telehealth
University of Oulu
P.O. Box 5000
90014 Oulu
Finland

Kurt Schicho
Medical University of Vienna
University Hospital of Cranio-Maxillofacial and Oral Surgery
Waehringer Guertel 18–20
1090 Vienna
Austria

Franco Servadei
Neurosurgical Unit "Hub & Spoke" PARMA-REGGIO EMILIA
Emergency Department
University Hospital of Parma
Viale Gramsci 14, 43100 Parma
Italy

James E. Silberzweig
Department of Radiology
St. Luke's-Roosevelt Hospital Center
1000 Tenth Avenue
New York, NY 10019
USA

Fernanda Tagliaferri
Intensive Care Unit
M. Bufalini Hospital
47023 Cesena
Italy

Pierre Vieyres
Laboratoire Vision & Robotique
University of Orléans
IUT de Bourges
63 avenue de Lattre de Tassigny
18020 Bourges Cedex
France

Davis Viprakasit
Department of Urology
Northwestern Memorial Hospital
675 N. St. Clair, Galter 20–150
Chicago, IL 60611
USA

Ernest Wang
Department of Neurosurgery
National Neuroscience Institute, Singapore
11 Jalan Tan Tock Seng
Singapore 308433
Singapore

Vahid Yaghmai
Northwestern Memorial Hospital
676 North St. Clair Street, Suite 800
Chicago, IL 60611-2927
USA

Jianguo Zhang
Shanghai Institute of Technical Physics
Chinese Academy of Sciences
Shanghai 200083
China

Abbreviations

ACR	American College of Radiology
ADO	ActiveX data object
ADSL	Asymmetric digital subscriber line
AH	Authentication header
AHLTA	Armed Forces Health Longitudinal Technology Application
AMEDD	Army Medical Department
ANN	Artificial neural networks
API	Application programming interface
APPMO	US Army PACS Program Management Office
ASP	Active server pages
ATNA	Audit trial and node authentication
ATP	Arizona Telemedicine Program
AVM	Arteriovenous malformation
bpp	Bits per pixel
CABG	Coronary artery bypass grafting
CALIC	Context-based adaptive lossless image codec
CAVELib	CAVE library
CAVE™	Cave automatic virtual environment
CCD	Charge-coupled device
CCF	Carotid cavernous fistula
CD	Compact disc
CDMA	Code division multiple access
CIR	Committed information rate
CME	Continuous medical education
COM	Component object model
CR	Compression ratio
CR	Computed radiography
CRT	Cathode ray tube
CSH	Combat support hospital

CT	Computed tomography
CTN	Central test node
C-Wall	Configurable wall
2D	Two-dimensional
3D	Three-dimensional
DCT	Discrete cosine transform
DICOM	Digital imaging and communications in medicine
DIN	Digital Imaging Network
DLL	Data link layer
DLP	Digital light processing
DoD	Department of Defense
DSL	Digital subscriber lines
DTRS	Deployable teleradiology system
EAP	Extensible authentication protocol
ECALIC	Enhanced CALIC
EHRS	Electronic health-care record system
e-mail	Electronic mail
EPR	Electronic patient record
ESCSH	English-speaking countries of the Southern Hemisphere
ESP	Encapsulating security payload
EUA	Enterprise user authentication
EVDO	Evolution Data Optimized
FCC	Federal Communications Commission
FinOHTA	Finnish Office for Health Technology Assessment
GATS	General Agreement on Trade in Services
GCS	Glasgow Coma Scale
GDP	Gross domestic product
GH	General hospital
GIF	Graphics Interchange Format
GSM	Global system for mobile communication
GUI	Graphical user interface
HIS	Hospital information system
H-O	Heckscher–Ohlin
HSDPA	High-Speed Downlink Pocket Access
HTTP	Hypertext transfer protocol
HTTPS	Hypertext transfer protocol over secure socket layer

ICD	International Classification of Diseases
ICMPv6	Internet control message protocol for Internet protocol version 6
ICT	Information and communication technology
ICU	Intensive care unit
IEEE	Institute of Electrical and Electronics Engineers
IHE	Integrating Healthcare Enterprise
IIS	Internet information services
INMARSAT	International maritime satellite
IP	Internet protocol
IPHs	Intraparenchymal contusions and hematomas
IPSec	Internet protocol security
IPv4	Internet protocol version 4
IPv6	Internet protocol version 6
IRP	Interventional radiology procedures
ISAPI	Internet server application programming interface
ISDN	Integrated systems digital network
ITI	Information technology infrastructure
JPEG	Joint Photographic Experts Group
JSWG	Joint Services Working Group
KLH	Kuala Lumpur Hospital
LAN	Local-area network
LCD	Liquid crystal display
LEAP	Lightweight extensible authentication protocol
LHP	Lifetime Health Plan
LRMC	Landstuhl Regional Medical Center
MAC	Media access control
MASH	Mobile Army Surgical Hospital
MATMO	Medical Advanced Technologies Management Office
MCPHIE	Mass Customized Personal Health Information & Education
MDIS	Medical diagnostic imaging support
MEDCOM	Medical Command
MIME	Multipurpose Internet mail extension
MMS	Multimedia messaging service
MOMEDA	Mobile Medical Data
MR	Magnetic resonance
MRCP	Magnetic resonance cholangiopancreatography

MRI	Magnetic resonance imaging
MTF	Medical treatment facility
NH	Neurosurgical hospital
OEF	Operation Enduring Freedom
OFDM	Orthogonal frequency division multiplexing
OIF	Operation Iraqi Freedom
ORB	Object request broker
OSI	Open systems interconnection
OTELO	Mobile tele-echography using an ultra-light robot
PACC	Partition, aggregation, and conditional coding
PC	Personal computer
PDA	Personal data assistant
PDU	Protocol data unit
PEAP	Protected extensible authentication protocol
PROMODAS	Professional Mobile Data Systems
QEH	Queen Elizabeth Hospital
QoS	Quality of service
QUANTA	Quality of service adaptive networking toolkit
RCCS	Remote Clinical Communications System
RCM	Remote center of motion
RLE	Run-length encoding
ROI	Region of interest
S/MIME	Secure MIME
SA	Security association
SCP	Service class provider
SCU	Service class user
SMTP	Simple mail transfer protocol
SSID	Service set identifier
SSL	Secure socket layer
TATRC	Telemedicine and Advanced Technology Research Center
TBI	Traumatic brain injury
TC	Telephonic consultation
TCP	Transmission control protocol
TIFF	Tagged Image File Format
TLS	Transport-layer security
TMED	Telemedicine
TR	Teleradiology
tSAH	Traumatic subarachnoid hemorrhage

UIC	University of Illinois at Chicago
USAMRMC	US Army Medical Research and Materiel Command
UTM	Universiti Teknologi Malaysia
VA	Veterans administration
VC	Videocounseling
VGA	Video graphics array
VMP	Volume manipulation program
VPN	Virtual private network
VR	Virtual reality
VRMedLab	Virtual Reality in Medicine Lab
VSAT	Very small aperture terminal
WADO	Web access DICOM persistent object
WAN	Wide-area network
WCHM	WorldCare Health (Malaysia)
WEP	Wired equivalent privacy
Wi-Max	Worldwide Interoperative Microwave Access
Win32	Windows NT and Windows 95 and up
WLAN	Wireless local-area network
WPA	Wi-Fi protected access
WTO	World Trade Organization
XDS	Cross-enterprise document sharing
XDS-I	Cross-enterprise document sharing for images
XML	Extensible markup language

Introduction to Teleradiology

Sajeesh Kumar

Abstract Telemedicine aids in examination, investigation, monitoring, and treatment of patients who are located away from the physician. Teleradiology is a branch of telemedicine in which electronic transmission of radiological patient images, such as X-rays, computed tomography images, and magnetic resonance images, takes place. A basic teleradiology system consists of three major components: an image-sending station, a transmission network, and a receiving/image-review station. In addition to its vast application in medical fields, teleradiology can also be useful for training new radiologists, assisting and training radiologists in developing countries, diagnosing injured soldiers on or near the battlefield, performing radiological procedures in space, etc.

1.1
Introduction to Telemedicine

Telemedicine is a method by which patients can be examined, investigated, monitored, and treated, with the patient and the physician being located at different places. *Tele* is a Greek word meaning "distance," and *mederi* is a Latin word meaning "to heal". Although initially considered "futuristic" and "experimental," telemedicine is today a reality and has come to stay. In telemedicine one transfers the expertise, not the patient. Hospitals of the future will drain patients from all over the world without geographical limitations. High-quality medical services can be brought to the patient, rather than transporting the patient to distant and expensive tertiary-care centers. A major goal of telemedicine is to eliminate unnecessary traveling of patients and their escorts. Image acquisition, image storage, image display and processing, and image transfer represent the basis of telemedicine. Telemedicine is becoming an integral part of health-care services in several countries.

1.2
What Is Teleradiology

Teleradiology is the electronic transmission of radiological patient images, such as X-rays, computed tomography (CT) images, and magnetic resonance images, from one location to another for the purposes of interpretation and/or consultation. Typically, this is done over standard telephone lines, a wide-area network, or a local-area network. Through teleradiology, images can be sent to another part of the hospital or to other locations around the world. The word "teleradiology" (pronunciation, "tel-&-"rAd-E-'äl-&-jE) is derived from the Greek word *tele*, meaning "far off," and "radiology," meaning "the use of radiation (such as X-rays) or other imaging technologies (such as ultrasound and magnetic resonance imaging) to diagnose or treat disease."

Teleradiology is a branch of telemedicine in which telecommunication systems are used to transmit radiological images from one location to another. The earliest effort in teleradiology probably dates back to 1929 when dental X-rays were transmitted over telegraph to a distant location [2]. An initial attempt in using the Web in an emergency medical situation describes the use of digital cameras to take clinical photographs and scanners to scan radiographs, with conversion of the resulting digital images to a JPEG format using Adobe Photoshop and then transmission via the Internet [1]. Today, digitized images are transmitted around the globe, via high-speed telecommunication links, on a regular basis.

1.2.1
Acquisition of Images

Today, virtually all radiology equipments are fully DICOM compliant. Thus, images can be stored on a network or a workstation in the DICOM format. Lossy and lossless compressions are possible, with varying degrees of loss of information, which may be acceptable depending on the modality and the clinical situation. Plain radiographs obtained nondigitally may need to be scanned. Currently, mammography images remain the last barrier to reliable teleradiology, owing to the large file sizes and issues related to the image resolution required to detect microcalcifications.

1.2.2
Transfer of Images

In the early days, transfer of images was performed over telephone lines using modems, sometimes with speeds as low as 2,400 bps. Today, high-speed lines are available, allowing different centers to connect directly or over the Internet, for transmission of images. Images may be directly transferred or streamed, depending on the software being used.

1.2.3
Viewing of Images

Image viewing requires a workstation that can display high-resolution images. Many software programs are currently available, e.g., EFilm, which allow viewing, manipulation, measurements, three-dimensional reconstructions, etc. The viewing software should allow reporting and storage, and transmission of the reports as well.

1.3
Basic System Components

A basic teleradiology system consists of three major components:

1. An image-sending station
2. A transmission network
3. A receiving/image review station

Patient images are electronically encoded in a digital format at the sending station, sent on the transmission network, and received, viewed, and possibly stored at the review station.

1.3.1
Image-Sending Station

The image-sending station consists of:

- An image (film) digitizer
- A network interface device (most commonly a phone modem)

Once the film digitizer has converted the image into a digital format, the data are sent to the modem upon command of the equipment operator. The modem is the control device, which converts digital data into electrical impulses that are sent along the transmission network.

The three most important specifications for a teleradiology sending station are resolution, compression, and transmission speed.

1.3.1.1
Image Resolution

Resolution is the ability of an imaging system to differentiate among objects. When a sending station digitizes an X-ray film, it breaks it into a two-dimensional matrix of small elements called pixels.

As the image is read by the digitizer, the information contained in each pixel is assigned a number, which represents the amount (or density) of information it contains. This number is called the gray-scale (or density) number. A pixel that has a lot of formation (black) would be assigned a higher number than a pixel with little information (light). The more the pixels in an image and the greater the range of density numbers per pixel, the better the image resolution.

1.3.1.2
Compression

Compression is a software technique by which certain pixels in the digitized image are dropped to decrease transmission time. Compression is expressed as a ratio. A compression ratio of 10:1 means that for each pixel of information retained from the original digitized matrix, ten pixels have been dropped before transmission. Compression algorithms below about 3:1 are usually considered lossless; that is, no information contained in the original digitized image is lost. Compression ratios above this are considered lossy (destructive) and can result in image degradation.

1.3.1.3
Transmission (Modem) Speed

A modem is the interface unit between the image digitizer and the transmission network. It converts digital image data to electrical impulses, which can be sent along the transmission media. The rate at which a modem can perform this conversion is given in bits per second.

The ideal teleradiology sending station would have very high resolution, little or no compression, and very high transmission speeds. This is not possible in the real world because optimizing one parameter negatively affects another (e.g., increasing resolution matrix size increases transmission time). How does one select a teleradiology sending unit to balance resolution, compression, and transmission speed parameters? If economically feasible, one selects a sending station that has a reasonably fast modem, an operator-selectable resolution of 512–2,048 bits, and several selectable compression levels. A station with this flexibility will allow the sender (and receiver) to decide on a case-by-case basis which is more important, quality of the received image, or the speed at which it arrives. If selectable resolution and compression are not an option, the sending station should have a reasonably high fixed resolution and lossless compression (3:1).

1.3.2
Transmission Network

The transmission network can be wire, fiber optics, or microwave. The most commonly used transmission networks currently in use for teleradiology are those provided by the telephone companies. Such networks utilize both wire and fiber optics. Transmission speeds (and cost) are closely related to the transmission mode.

1.3.3
Receiving/Image-Review Station

A receiving/image-review station consists of four broad categories:(1) modem, (2) computer hardware, (3) image-enhancement software, and (4) monitor(s).

1.3.3.1
Modem

The modem's maximum speed (baud rate) influences the data transmission time of the teleradiology sending station. To maintain maximum transmission speed, the receiving unit must be equipped with a modem of maximum speed equal to or greater than that of the sending station.

1.3.3.2
Computer Hardware

The specification parameters for teleradiology applications are the same as for general computing applications. The computer hard disk is used to store the received images.

Teleradiology systems store data in either a noncompressed or a compressed format.

1.3.3.3
Image-Enhancement Software

Most teleradiology systems have gray-scale window/level and magnification image-enhancement software. These should be included in any teleradiology system considered for purchase. Other software enhancement features that may be included are color, gray-scale mapping, positive–negative reversal, annotation, minification, edge enhancement, image flip/rotate, cine, and histogram equalization. The value of these additional software enhancements is subjective and largely dependent on the types of images viewed and the preference of the radiologists using the review station.

1.3.3.4
Monitors

The most common specifications stated for teleradiology monitors are monitor resolution and screen size. Resolutions range from approximately 512 × 512 to 2,048 × 2,048 pixels. It is generally recommended that for teleradiology applications, monitors have a pixel resolution of 1,000 × 1,000 or above. Monitor screen sizes generally range from 14 to 21 in. The larger monitors provide a better viewing environment.

Two other monitor specifications might be considered when purchasing a teleradiology system:

1. Split screen
2. Monitor (CRT) brightness

Split-screen capability is a feature that allows the display of two or more different images on the monitor at the same time. This feature is important if two images need to be compared by the radiologist.

Monitor brightness is the specification for the maximum intensity of white light that a CRT can display. It is usually given in units of footlambert. This information is seldom given in vendor specifications but is important when comparing teleradiology viewing stations. Brighter monitors (with high footlambert values) are better for viewing because the brightness differential between the shades is greater and thus easier for the human eye to detect.

1.4
Scope of Teleradiology

Users of teleradiology systems include the following:

■ *Radiologists on call*: In this application, the on-call radiologist uses a portable teleradiology receiving station at home. Patient images are transmitted from the hospital (or clinic) to the physician's home for immediate review. This allows instantaneous consultation of the radiologist with the referring physician. Intensive care patient images taken in the Radiology Department can be quickly transmitted for review by the health-care team.

- *Hospital physicians:* Intensive care unit (ICU) patient images taken in the Radiology Department can be quickly transmitted to the ICU for review by the team responsible for that patient's care. Physicians or other health-care providers at other sites, who are involved in the care of an individual patient, can also view the images.
- *Primary-care and rural physicians:* A rural primary-care physician can send patient images taken in the clinic to a radiologist at a distant location for reading and consultation.
- *Physicians requiring remote subspecialty radiology consultations:* A community-hospital radiologist can send a complete set of images to a remote radiologist who is a subspecialist (e.g., pediatric radiologist).

Potential applications of teleradiology also include:

- Training new radiologists
- Assisting and training radiologists in developing countries
- Diagnosing injured soldiers on or near the battlefield
- Performing radiological procedures in space
- Collaborating and mentoring during radiology by radiologists around the globe

1.5
Relevance of Teleradiology in Developing Countries

Ideally, every citizen in the world should have immediate access to the appropriate specialist for medical consultation. However, the current status of the health service is such that total medical care cannot be provided in rural areas. Even secondary and tertiary medical care is not uniformly available in suburban and urban areas. Incentives to entice specialist radiologists to practice in suburban or rural areas have failed in many nations.

It is generally considered that the communities most likely to benefit from teleradiology are those least likely to be able to afford it or to have the requisite communication infrastructure. However, this may no longer be true. In contrast to the bleak scenario in health care, Internet connections and computer literacy are developing fast and prices are falling. Theoretically, it is far easier to set up an excellent telecommunication infrastructure in suburban and rural areas than to place hundreds of medical specialists in these places. The world has realized that the future of telecommunications lies in satellite-based technology and fiber-optic cables. Providing health care in remote areas using high technology is not as absurd as it may initially appear. Could even the greatest optimist have anticipated the phenomenal explosion in the use of computers in the villages of India?

1.6
Rewards of Teleradiology

Worldwide, there is difficulty in retaining radiologists in nonurban areas. Once the virtual presence of a radiologist is acknowledged through teleradiology, a patient can access resources in a tertiary radiological center without the constraints of distance. Teleradiology also ensures maximal utilization of suburban or rural hospitals. Teleradiology may also avoid unnecessary travel and expense for the patient and the families and improves health outcomes.

It is also personally and professionally rewarding to know that each of us has played a role to increase access to radiological services and to improve quality of care. Few moments are as rewarding as receiving an anxious look from a patient in need and giving reassurances that access to the best care is only a moment away.

Summary

- Telemedicine aids in examination, investigation, monitoring, and treatment of patients who are located away from the physician.
- Teleradiology is a branch of telemedicine in which electronic transmission of radiological patient images, such as X-rays, CT images, and magnetic resonance images, takes place.
- A basic teleradiology system consists of three major components: an image-sending station, a transmission network, and a receiving/image-review station.
- In addition to its vast application in medical fields, teleradiology can also be useful for training new radiologists, assisting and training radiologists in developing countries, diagnosing injured soldiers on or near the battlefield, performing radiological procedures in space, etc.

References

1. Johnson D, Goel R, Paul B, Hirst P (1998) Transferring medical images on the world wide web for emergency clinical management: a case report. BMJ 316:988–989
2. (1929) Sending dental X-rays by telegraph. Dent Radiogr Photogr 2:16

The Future of Teleradiology in Medicine Is Here Today

Brad C. Hearaly, Davis Viprakasit, and William K. Johnston III

Abstract Teleradiology is transferring of medical images through an Internet provider from a primary system to a remote location. Compressed digital imaging tools and the picture archiving and communication system have helped teleradiology to become more accessible and feasible to physicians. Wireless transmission using portable viewers has the potential to further improve its application and accessibility. In order to protect confidential medical records from being accessible to unauthorized individuals, security measures such as the establishment of a virtual private network between hospitals and receiving locations have been taken. Teleradiology provides students, residents, and even attending physicians with access to a limitless number of images for reference from almost anywhere in the world and helps improve their continued exposure and experience in the health-care setting.

2.1
Introduction

Teleradiology is the practice of transferring medical images electronically through an Internet provider from a primary system to a remote location for the diagnosis or treatment of patients. With the widespread availability of the Internet today, the sharing of medical imaging between physicians has become more commonplace. Smaller medical practices in rural communities can now share knowledge and resources with larger health-care providers in urban settings without changing locations. Magnetic resonance images, computed tomography (CT) images, angiograms, and even classical X-rays can be transferred electronically in a matter of seconds to minutes from one health provider to another. As a result, medical images can easily be shared within the same facility, between facilities of the same practice, between physicians of different practices, or even from the hospital to the home of a physician via a computer. Furthermore, consulting and treating physicians can access films at any location with

Internet connections, and, with the growing availability of wireless Internet, teleradiology access has become nearly unlimited. While physicians of all medical specialties may soon incorporate some aspect of the field into their daily work, currently radiologists most commonly utilize teleradiology in their practice. In order to demonstrate the use of teleradiology, the American College of Radiology (ACR) poled radiologists in the years 1999 and 2003 to determine how prevalent the use of teleradiology was among radiologists [4]. The data showed an increase in use over time from 1999 to 2003. There were also significant differences between the types of practices and the use of teleradiology. Academic practices, rural-setting practices, and practices with a larger number of radiologists tended to utilize teleradiology at a higher prevalence than other practices. From these data, one can infer that teleradiology is a significant advancement used in education and to improve patient care.

2.2
History: The Beginning

With the advent of the Internet in the early 1990s, teleradiology was born. One of the primary obstacles in the development of teleradiology was the conversion of analogue images into digital formats, in order to facilitate the transfer of images via the Internet. Before the digital age of the digital versatile disk, medical images were primarily stored in analogue format [physical quantity (electric)]. In order to transmit these pictures via the Internet, these images needed to be converted to a digital binary code [(0,1)]. The primary problem with digital conversion was that these documents occupied a large amount of pixel storage and size. In order to have maximum resolution and to provide clear pictures, the images require a great number of pixels, which in turn results in larger file sizes and corresponding transmission times. For example, the ACR recommends that small matrix size radiographs (such as from MRI, CT, ultrasound nuclear medicine, digital fluorography, and digitized radiographic films) should provide a minimum matrix size of 512×512 (0.26 megapixels) at a minimum 8-bit pixel depth (color depth). Similarly, ACR recommendations for large matrix size radiographs (including those from digital radiography and digitized radiographic films, i.e., scanned X-rays) should provide a minimum of 2.51 pixel/mm special resolution (approximately 4.0 megapixels) at a minimum of 10-bit pixel depth [2]. Thus, scanned X-ray files can be quite massive and exceed 1 MB in size. This creates transfer difficulties when the standard Internet connections can only maximally upload a file at a speed of less than 1 kbps. This would require 30 min to upload one image at a time and an additional 20 min to download the image from the Internet to a remote computer.

In order to overcome long transfer times, image compression of digitalized files into a Joint Photographic Experts Group (JPEG) file or Graphics Interchange Format (GIF) was devised. JPEG and GIF files are typically compressed at ratios of 20:1 and 10:1, respectively [15], without losing any resolution. Thus, digital images can be compressed in JPEG format or GIF down to more manageable sizes of 20–100 kB, respectively, and this leads to a decrease in subsequent transfer times.

In addition to the creation of compressed digital imaging tools, the development of the picture archiving and communication system (PACS) has also helped circumvent the analogue to digital problem in the storage of medical images. The PACS allows digital storage of medical images, thus making the transfer of images to a remote location much more efficient and eliminating the need for analogue file conversion. Today, magnetic resonance images, CT, images, angiograms, and ultrasound images are now all commonly stored in a digital format directly into the PACS. In addition, plain X-ray films are similarly stored in a digital format with the PACS to avoid scanning analogue films into a digital format.

2.3
Future Goals and Benefits

The contributions of compressed digital imaging tools and the PACS have allowed the field of teleradiology to become more accessible and feasible to physicians. Given the wide array of potential uses, the ACR has established goals for incorporating teleradiology into daily medical practice. With each goal, a potential benefit to the radiologist and other treating physicians exists. These goals are primarily focused on improving patient care through an increased networking among physicians in order to reach a conclusive diagnosis (Table 2.1).

2.4
Technical Framework: Backbone for Teleradiology

The technical framework of the Internet serves as the backbone for teleradiology. The rate-limiting step in teleradiology is the speed at which data can be transferred. In 1990, the first medical images were sent via a dial-up service over standard phone lines at the University of Kansas Medical Center [13]. At that time, the maximum capabilities of the dial-up server were download speeds of 56 kbps over a standard phone line. Soon after, the new technology of digital subscriber lines (DSL), initially developed by Joe Lechleider of Bellcore in 1988, began to have increased utility in data transfer. DSL increased the

Table 2.1. A list of goals set forth by the American College of Radiology (*ACR*) for the advancement of teleradiology and the benefits of each [2]

ACR goals for teleradiology	Benefits
1. Provide access for consultation and interpretation of films from peripheral locations	Allow for second opinions from physicians at offsite locations and/or opinions from subspecialties of radiology
2. Provide radiologic support in health facilities without a radiologist	Underserved rural communities gain access to radiologists throughout the world
3. Provide immediate radiologic image interpretation for both nonemergent and emergent patient care	Saves time and decreases the risk of misplacing or losing images by avoiding mailing hard copies of images. Furthermore, the radiologist can access images from home computers, PDAs, or even phones to provide information back to treating physicians
4. Return interpreted images back to referring providers	Interpreted images are efficiently returned to the primary-care or emergency-room physician
5. Improved interpretation	Traveling imaging centers can relay their information directly to a major medical center where image reading can be overlooked by a number of physicians. This will decrease the time needed to interpret images in addition to decreasing the number of misdiagnosed patients owing to error with image interpretation
6. Teleradiology supports telemedicine	Instead of explaining an image or finding, the image can be sent directly to a corresponding physician
7. Sharing and availability enhance educational for practicing radiologists	As new information and data come out, it will be more efficient for physicians to become educated via image transfer with teleradiology

PDA personal digital assistant

speed of data transfer by relying on existing copper phone lines and now provide maximum rates of 6.0 Mbps [3]. Although traditional voice signals travel over phone lines on a very limited range of frequencies, local telephone cables can carry signals at frequencies well above and below the frequencies used for phone calls. DSL use the advantage of these unused frequencies to transmit data. In the mid-1990s, the new development of cable broadband became available and pushed data transfer rates even faster (currently a maximum of 30 Mbps) [11]. The drawback to cable Internet is that it is a "shared" network, and multiple subscribers are feeding from the same source. Thus, during peak usage, cable Internet providers do not provide transfer speeds anywhere near their advertised capabilities. More recently, the advent of bundled copper lines came into use with T1 and T3 cables. The advertised speed capabilities with these modalities are up to 1.5 Mbps [3] for T1 connections, and newer T3 cables allowed speeds of 45 Mbps [3]. Thus, using a T3 broadband at a speed of 45 Mbps, one can upload and transmit a CT scan with a size of 100 Mb in only 2.2 s. Although fast, this transfer rate is well below the maximum capabilities of 9.08 Gbps, which would make transmission nearly instantaneous (University of Tokyo) [9]. These speeds are accomplished via fiber-optic technology, which uses a thin glass tube and light impulses to propagate a signal. These light impulses have much higher speed capabilities than the previously mentioned copper wire connections. Therefore, newer technologies are continually being sought to increase the speed of data transfer.

The most recent development in data transfer tools has been the use of wireless technology. In the early 1990s, wireless data transfer began to surface, and in 1995 Yamamoto [17] reported the first use of wireless radiologic data transfer. Wireless networks use both radiofrequency and microwaves for data transfer as opposed to hard-wired lines composed of copper or fiber-optic cables. The most common form of wireless network can be found at local coffee shops and airports and is referred to as a wireless local-area network, which conforms to the 802.11 Wi-Fi standards (microwave frequency) [5]. The signals used by wireless Internet connections are similar to that used in cellular phones. Cellular phones transmit radiofrequency signals to a base tower, which in turn can relay the signal. Different frequencies are used to send a signal back to the phone from the tower to limit interference. These "wireless" signals are ultimately linked to the hard-line phone network by base towers that relay data directly to the hard-wired network (fiber optic or copper). Thus, the wireless network is composed of both radio and microwave signals, which are connected to hard-wired lines by large (cellular network) or small antennas. With the advent of wireless technology, the current maximum data transfer speed of 72 Mbps [current potential of Worldwide Interoperative Microwave Access (Wi-Max) technology] [17] is dramatically faster than the 56 kbps achieved over standard phone lines. However, typical of all wireless technology, the maximum data stream is a function of distance from the nearest base station. Therefore, the maximum speeds of Wi-Max and other wireless technology [Evolution Data Optimized (EVDO) and High-Speed Downlink Pocket Access (HSDPA)] are not representative of their practical capabilities.

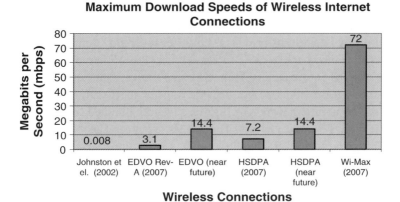

Fig. 2.1. Download capabilities of past, present, and future wireless Internet connections. The Cingular network is very metropolitan based and the Wi-Max network basically is a work in progress in the USA (started in Russia)

Wireless transmission using portable viewers has the potential to further improve the application and accessibility of teleradiology. In 2005, Johnston et al. [10] demonstrated that images of renal colic with obstructing kidney stones or renal trauma cases could be transmitted through a simple wireless personal data assistant (PDA) connection and received for interpretation [16]. The download capability of wireless at that time was only 1 kbps (PDA through phone). However, download speeds have become faster as the technology in portable wireless units has improved. The new HSDPA (Cingular Wireless, Chicago, IL, USA) is capable of reaching download speeds of 7.2 Mbps (Fig. 2.1) [7]. This 3G technology was recently released in 2005 and is the first wireless technology that allows simultaneous voice and data streams. By providing separate channels for data transfer, the downloading of a Web page on the data stream is not interrupted by the voice stream if there is an incoming call. Presently, HSDPA is only available in 18 large metropolitan markets in the USA. Code Division Multiple Access–EVDO, a more commonly available 3G technology (Sprint and Verizon), was released in the USA in 2002, and is the primary wireless access found in urban settings across the world (Europe and Asia). Recently, EVDO-carrying companies have been upgrading to an EVDO Rev A product, which can match the speeds of HSDPA and also offers simultaneous voice and data streams. Further applications of teleradiology can be expected as the improvements in portable wireless units maximize the potential data transfer rates already achieved by wireless signaling.

In addition, portable wireless viewers may also use mobile satellite providers, such as Inmarnet's Broadband Global Area Network, for data signaling. Using satellite providers, global data coverage in wireless signaling is almost limitless with only small deficiencies in coverage at the polar ice caps [8]. The maximum download speed for some satellite providers is approximately 2 Mbps [1]. Unfortunately, like any satellite technology, weather can interfere with the signal transmitted to and from the receiver, thus decreasing expected download speeds.

2.5
Teleradiology Security and Preservation of Confidentiality: How Health Providers Maintain Confidentiality with the Electronic Transmission of Patient Records

The issue of patient confidentiality and Internet security arises whenever medical data are sent over the Internet. Because of the concern that unauthorized individuals may be able to obtain access to confidential medical records during transmission, a secure connection must be established from hospitals to the external remote location. Currently, the most widely used security measure among teleradiology services involves the establishment of a virtual private network (VPN) between hospitals and receiving locations [14]. A VPN provides a secure connection via the Internet, which mimics a private point-to-point connection. Employees on the road or at home may connect in a secure fashion to the corporate network via public access. All images and data sent over a VPN are encrypted. In order for physicians to decipher and view the medical images, they must enter a code from an encryption key that is personalized to each physician. Each key is updated and changed frequently. Therefore, data intercepted by hackers on a public or shared network are not interpretable unless they have access granted through the encryption keys. For security reasons, a VPN must also provide audit and accounting records to show who has accessed what information at what time. In doing so, medical images, as well as medical information, can be sent in a secure manner over a public network with verification of the intended viewer.

2.6
Education and Training: Increasing the Knowledge of Physicians with Increased Image Exposure

The ability for physicians to share images quickly and cost-effectively over the Internet allows for the continuing education throughout the medical community. Teleradiology provides students, residents, and even attending physicians with access to a limitless number of images for reference from almost anywhere in the world. Health-care providers treating rarer medical ailments have the ability to utilize the data banks or physicians' expertise from more endemic areas. In doing so, all physicians can improve their continued exposure and experience in the health-care setting and further develop subspecialized areas of interest or expertise if desired without changing locations. For example, a radiologist could become an expert in reading hand films. He or she may receive inquiries via teleradiology for consultations, second opinion, and/or confirmation of prior interpretations from a physician with less experience in hand pathology. As a result of this interaction, both physicians will benefit—either by gaining more experience with specialized diseases or by direct expert opinion in nonendemic areas.

2.7
Future Directions: Where Wireless Communications Could Take Teleradiology

Wireless connections are becoming increasingly available throughout the world. Satellite broadband is accessible in most countries and access plans through cellular phone providers are not far behind. In 2007, the number of cellular phone users passed the three billion mark [6]. In addition to availability, the speed of wireless technology is ever-increasing. Once a technology reaches its maximum capability, another technology appears to replace it. Once EVDO and HSDPA reach their respectable maximum download speeds (Fig. 2.1) [7, 12], the new technology Wi-Max (4G technology) will likely be out of its infant stage and have increased availability throughout the world. Wi-Max is a new wireless technology service being adapted by most industrialized nations. It is similar to Wi-Fi (common wireless networks at coffee shops, colleges, and airports), with the added ability to be broadcast over a much larger area of interest (up to 30 miles). For example, Korea Telecom is in the process of deploying its version of Wi-Max (WiBro) throughout the entire city of Seoul, South Korea. Its network will assist in the signal control of subway transportation and has speeds of up to 1–3 Mbps. Intel (via Australia's Unwired) and Sprint/Nextel have already predicted that Wi-Max will eventually replace many hard-wired communication services with upper limits of Wi-Max Internet connection of 72 Mbps (Fig. 2.1).

Overall, the primary goal of teleradiology is to provide improved health care to patients by expediting disease diagnoses with quicker and more specialized interpretations of medical images and data. In addition, physicians will have more exposure to large databases of radiological images in which to familiarize themselves, in order to bring the best possible diagnostic skills to patients. Wireless teleradiology will aid in the treatment of emergency cases or when a specific specialist must be reached outside of the work place both locally and worldwide. Health-care providers in remote regions of the world with poor hard-line Internet capabilities will benefit most from wireless teleradiology, by bridging potential deficiencies in medical image interpretations and consultations. Despite increased resources, even industrialized countries will benefit from wireless teleradiology, as certain modalities such as MRI are not readily available at every hospital and a traveling MRI machine must be utilized for nonemergency patients. Wireless broadband would be ideal for these machines, if a situation arises when interpretation must be made from a remote location. Thus, wireless teleradiology can bridge the gap and better equalize health-care knowledge in all different settings.

2.8
Conclusion

The ability to transmit information worldwide through an almost instantaneous Internet connection is before us today. Teleradiology allows the sharing of medical images between different health-care professionals and improves care of patients. Its role in medicine will increase exponentially as transmission speeds continue to improve.

Summary

- Teleradiology is transferring of medical images through an Internet provider from a primary system to a remote location.
- Compressed digital imaging tools and the PACS have helped teleradiology to become more accessible and feasible to physicians. Wireless transmission using portable viewers has the potential to further improve its application and accessibility.
- In order to protect confidential medical records from being accessible to unauthorized individuals, security measures such as the establishment of a VPN between hospitals and receiving locations have been taken.
- Teleradiology provides students, residents, and even attending physicians with access to a limitless number of images for reference from almost anywhere in the world and helps improve their continued exposure and experience in the health-care setting.
- The primary goal of teleradiology is to provide improved health care to patients by expediting disease diagnoses with quicker and more specialized interpretations of medical images and data.

References

1. Agristar Global Networks. Overview. http://www.agristar.com/agristar400.shtml. Last Accessed date 30 April 2008
2. American College of Radiology. ACR standard for teleradiology. http://imaging.stryker.com/images/ACR_Standards-Teleradiology.pdf
3. Broad band info.com. Compare T1, T3, and DSL connections. http://www.broadbandinfo.com/internet-access/dsl/t1-t3-compare.html
4. Ebbert TL, Meghea C, Iturbe S, Forman HP, Bhargavan M, Sunshine JH (2007) The state of teleradiology in 2003 and changes since 1999. Am J Radiol 188:W103–W112
5. How Mobile Phone Networks Work (2001). http://www.sitefinder.ofcom.org.uk/mobilework.htm
6. http://en.wikipedia.org/wiki/Evdo
7. http://en.wikipedia.org/wiki/HSDPA
8. Inmarsat. http://www.inmarsat.com/Services/Land/BGAN/Coverage.aspx?language=EN&textonly=False
9. Internet 2 land speed record. http://www.internet2.edu/lsr
10. Johnston WK III, Patel BN, Low RK, Das S (2005) Wireless teleradiology for renal colic and renal trauma. J Endourol 19:32–36
11. Mitchell B. DSL vs cable - broadband Internet speed comparison. http://compnetworking.about.com/od/dslvscablemodem/a/speedcompare.htm
12. Ridley K. Global mobile phone use to pass 3 billion. Reuters. http://uk.reuters.com/article/technologyNews/idUKL2712199720070627
13. Templeton AW, Dwyer SJ, Rosenthal SJ, Eckard DA, Harrison LA, Cook LT (1991) A dial-up digital teleradiology system: technical considerations and clinical experience. Am J Roentgenol 157(6):1331–1336
14. Virtual private networking: an overview. http://www.microsoft.com/technet/prodtechnol/windows2000serv/plan/vpnoverview.mspx
15. Webreference (2000) Compression: optimizing web graphics. http://www.webreference.com/dev/graphics/compress.html
16. WiMax (2007) Mobile mentalism. http://mobilementalism.com/2007/04/21/nokia-to-release-70 mbps-phones-next-year/
17. Yamamoto LG (1995) Wireless teleradiology and fax using cellular phones and notebook PCs for instant access to consultants. Am J Emerg Med 13(2):184–187

Compression of Medical Images for Teleradiology

Rajasvaran Logeswaran

Abstract Compression is necessary for storage and transmission of the large number of radiologic images in hospitals. Many lossless and lossy compression algorithms are available. Good lossy compression has statistically no observable difference from lossless compression. A study shows that lossy compression may be beneficial for diagnosis. Modeling provides better visualization and good lossy compression.

3.1
Background Information

Radiology plays a vital role in modern diagnosis, through the various non-invasive and minimally invasive medical images it produces. Through the years, diagnostic imaging technology has evolved to produce images of almost every part of the body, even at the cellular and functional levels (e.g., functional magnetic resonance imaging, MRI) and at ever-increasing resolutions. Unlike the traditional X-ray (or roentgenology), where often only a single image or film is stored, modern radiologic imaging often produces a multitude of images per patient per examination.

As an example, a certain sequence of MRI, known as magnetic resonance cholangiopancreatography (MRCP) for the pancreatobiliary structures in the liver and abdominal regions, often produces 100–200 images per patient during a single examination. This usually start offs with the initial orientation or location of MRI images to position the liver and specifically the biliary tract (used to produce and transport bile that is used in digestion, absorption of fat-soluble vitamins and minerals, and removal of fat-soluble waste products such as cholecterol) in the abdomen. Several axial (horizontal slice) and coronal (vertical frontal slice) images would be taken. Both T1- and T2-weighted sequences, each highlighting different characteristics, may be taken for better visualization. This is followed by thick slab images (e.g., a volume 50 mm thick) to focus on the region of interest (ROI). Acquisitions from different angles may also be made and then the images are generated into a 3D reprojection of the ROI, to provide a pseudovolume representation. Thin-slice images (e.g., 8 mm thick or less) of the ROI are taken for more detailed study of the structures. Both T1- and T2-weighted sequences may be taken for these thin slices as well.

In many modalities, additional images with contrast agents are taken to highlight various parts or functions of interest. In some cases, the busy radiologist (medical specialist) may not be available at the time of image acquisition; thus, the radiographer (radiologic technologist) may acquire additional sets of images in order to ensure that the radiologist is presented with sufficient information and that the patient is not unduly discomforted by being subject to yet another examination for the lack of some information. This results in a large number of images generated and stored during a radiologic examination. Assuming an approximate image file size of 135 kB for a 256 × 256 pixels, 12 bits per pixel (bpp) image, which was the case for most of the MRI/MRCP images in the author's experience, approximately 15 MB of image data would be stored per examination. With just 50 examinations a day, over 250 GB of image data would be generated per year. This figure does not include images from other imaging modalities, such as computed tomography (CT), ultrasound, positron emission tomography, single photon emission CT, magnetic resonance spectroscopy, endoscopy, electroencephalogram, electrocardiogram, mammography, X-ray, and many more, which may be of higher resolution (typically 512 × 512 pixels) as well as multiple examinations (in one or more modalities) that the patient may go through in certain cases for difficult diagnosis. Also, for legal and diagnostic reasons, most medical institutions would have to retain patient records for at least several years and sometimes even indefinitely. This easily generates hundreds of terabytes of data that have to be archived in the picture archiving and communication system (PACS) [9] of the hospital information system of a medical institution over the years.

Although technology may be advancing rapidly in developing larger amounts of storage for less cost and reduced required physical space (e.g., USB flash drives 2 in. long can now store up to 10 GB of data), it is inevitable that the imaging equipment as well as paperless hospital systems generate an ever-increasing amount of digital data to be stored. As such, effective schemes are necessary for keeping the data size manageable, especially for the purposes of archiving and transmission.

Compression is essentially the representation of information using less space through removal of redundancies or reorganization of the data patterns in a more compact manner. Generally, there are two types of compression, namely, lossless and lossy [4]. In lossless (or reversible) compression, the compressed data can be completely restored to the original form with absolutely no loss of information. In lossy (or irreversible) compression, on the other hand, some of the less significant information is usually discarded during compression; thus, the restored data would not be a perfect match to the original data. However, a good lossy compression usually produces very little perceivable loss of information, as will be seen in Sect. 3.3. There are a host of popular compression techniques available for 2D and 3D images, both lossless and lossy. We will not go into the details of the algorithms in this chapter but merely mention the algorithms and some vital findings and give the references where the reader may, if desired, look up the relevant implementation and detailed studies conducted.

3.2
Global Experience with Reversible Compression

Although some digital radiology images may be stored in a variety of ways, for example, captured through an image grabber or video clip and stored as a conventional image file such as a Joint Photographic Experts Group (JPEG), Graphics Interchange Format, Tagged Image File Format, or bitmap, etc. file, a standard has been developed and is used in most PACS environments. This standard is known as digital imaging and communications in medicine (DICOM) [14], of which Part 10 of the standard relates to the DICOM file and media storage format that is used to store the medical images. The file format allows for a variable-length image header, with fields to incorporate information on the patient, radiologist, acquisition, parameter settings, annotations, image settings, and many others, in addition to the actual image data. Although many institutions store the radiology image as raw data in the DICOM files, the DICOM format does allow for several lossless and lossy compression schemes. Amongst these are variants of JPEG, JPEG-LS, and JPEG 2000 formats, run-length encoding (RLE), and Deflate (zip/gzip) [7]. In addition, many vendors tend to incorporate their own proprietary compression algorithms on such images as well.

As reported in [2], from a survey of coding, spatial and transform methods for 2D image compression, a compression system known as context-based adaptive lossless image codec (CALIC) [20] performed the best among the lossless algorithms tested. This technique used a gradient-based nonlinear predictor and arithmetic coding of symbols in different contexts, to produce better compression performance than the JPEG and JPEG-LS formats. An enhanced CALIC (ECALIC) [2] with better performance was developed, by improving on an adaptive binary mode, enhancing the error prediction, and introducing an adaptive histogram truncation scheme. The idea may be applicable in improving other prediction-based schemes as well. As for 3D images, it was shown in the same paper that a motion-based approach, incorporating ECALIC to compress the first image and subsequently using motion estimation, produced better results than the conventional wavelet-based techniques reported in [1, 18], and even some context-based techniques.

A good review on radiologic image compression is available in [19]. The paper provides evidence on the need for compression of radiologic images in storage and transmission and discusses several popular compression techniques. It is reported that entropy coding is not effective for radiologic images. Instead, popular compression techniques for these images reported in the literature concentrate on predictive and multiresolution models. The common lossless algorithms described in [19] include LZW, Huffman coding, arithmetic coding, RLE (mainly for images with low pixel variations, such as CT), differential pulse code modulation, hierarchical interpolation, difference pyramid, bit-plane encoding, and multiplicative autoregression. These are popular techniques that are described in most compression or information theory textbooks and in [19].

There are also many general-purpose lossless compression and archiving algorithms, such as bzip2 [17], which are known to produce good compression. These are applicable on generic image files, irrespective of the file format or information contained therein. As such, they can be valuable in preparing files for storage and transmission.

3.3
Global Experience with Irreversible Compression

Generally, medical experts (and regulatory institutions) are very reluctant to consider employing lossy (irreversible) compression to medical data, despite the obvious compression performance advantages, where the compression ratios (CRs) for this type of compression are usually several orders of magnitude higher than those of lossless compression of image and video data. The resistance to the lossy methods stems from the fear of loss of information resulting in loss of diagnostic quality of the images. However, reflecting on existing techniques, it is obvious that very often medical specialists put up with a lot of loss of information, such as in subsampling during image acquisition, without realizing it. Take, for example, the fact that in an ultrasound examination very few frames are captured and stored, even though the examination may last several minutes (hundreds of frames). In radiologic imaging, only selected images are acquired and stored, very often subject to a variety of losses in terms of acquisition artifacts, noise, bright spots, movement artifacts, nonoptimum orientations, partial volume effect, etc. Through experience, training, and familiarity with the images, radiologists are able to compensate for even large artifacts in images and still be comfortable in making a good diagnosis.

In recent times, there have been numerous research efforts supporting the viability of lossy compression for medical images. Take, for example, an MRI brain image shown in the top left of Fig. 3.1. In [3], it was reported that this

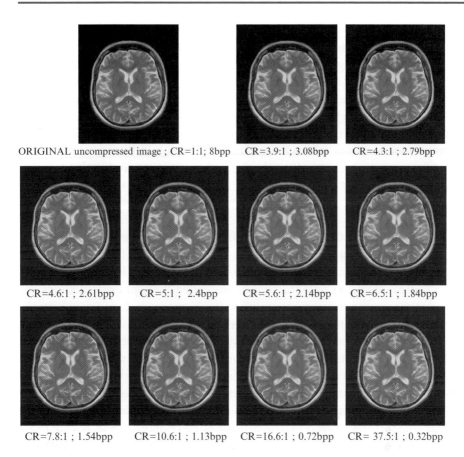

ORIGINAL uncompressed image ; CR=1:1; 8bpp   CR=3.9:1 ; 3.08bpp   CR=4.3:1 ; 2.79bpp

CR=4.6:1 ; 2.61bpp   CR=5:1 ; 2.4bpp   CR=5.6:1 ; 2.14bpp   CR=6.5:1 ; 1.84bpp

CR=7.8:1 ; 1.54bpp   CR=10.6:1 ; 1.13bpp   CR=16.6:1 ; 0.72bpp   CR= 37.5:1 ; 0.32bpp

Fig. 3.1. Magnetic resonance imaging brain image compressed progressively using lossy compression at different compression ratios (*CR*) and the corresponding resolution (bits per pixel)

8-bpp image was progressively compressed in a lossy manner up to a resolution of 0.32 bpp (i.e., an average of only 0.32 bits are used to represent each pixel's information), achieving a compression performance (measured in terms of CR) of up to 37.5:1. CR is the ratio of the original file size (S_O) to the final compressed size (S_C), or S_O/S_C. Thus, a CR of 37.5:1 means that the compressed file is only 1/37.5 times, or 2.7% of, the original file size. Even on close inspection of the images in the figure, there is very little observable difference between the various compressed images and the original image.

Studies such as that reported in [13] have shown that there was no significant difference (at the 95% confidence interval) in image quality and, more importantly, the diagnostic value between the tested uncompressed and controlled lossy compressed radiologic images. In [15], the authors proposed a possible protocol for evaluating the quality in various image modalities, with specific examples in lossy compressed digital mammograms. For images compressed using embedded wavelet at 0.15 bpp, their pilot study also showed that there was no statistically significant difference with the original analog images. Furthermore, it is well known that lossy techniques effect much greater compression than lossless compression. This fact is exploited by most popular image and video formats, which employ some amount of lossy compression to be able to deliver very high quality multimedia content on media with restricted storage capacity (e.g., VCD).

3.4
Education and Training: Benefits of Irreversible Compression and Modeling

It is of interest to note that image processing through lossy methods can sometimes improve diagnostic value as the human visual system is better, if not excellent, at filling in the "loss" more efficiently than filtering out distracting parts cluttered with wrong information (i.e., noise) that could influence it. Worse still, the distracting information can cause us to wrongly perceive the actual structures in the image. To illustrate this point, take the very simplified example below. The image on the left in Fig. 3.2 is corrupted by high-intensity (the white sections) foreign objects (e.g., noise). Studying the image, one may have several interpretations of what is represented. Upon having those unwanted objects removed, by truncating (thresholding) the high-intensity parts out, one obtains the actual image given on the right. In all likelihood, this resulting image is seen to be rather different from what was perceived of the original corrupted image. Also take note that although the resulting image

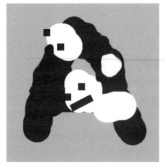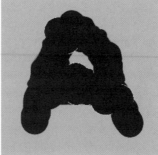

Fig. 3.2. Effect of beneficial lossy truncation on an image affected by noise

is not perfect, without the distracting information, our human visual system now can easily compensate for the imperfection and understand the image to represent the letter "A."

To test this theory, some studies were conducted for developing low-cost tele-medicine systems, which dealt with radiologic images. In one such study [14], a double-blind test was conducted amongst radiologists in the diagnostic imaging department, where the radiologists were asked to make their diagnosis on a set of randomly ordered medical images subjected to different levels of controlled lossy compression using the wavelet-based set partitioning in hierarchical trees algo-rithm [16]. The radiologists inevitably performed better with images subjected to the controlled lossy compression than they did with the original uncompressed images. Figure 3.3 shows a graph generated from the results of that study, where it is apparent that the accuracy of correct diagnosis was better at higher compression performance, as compared with the less compressed images.

A related study [5] showed that there was also no significant difference in using costly high-quality digitizers over conventional digital cameras to obtain digital versions of the medical images. Neither was there a significant difference in using high-resolution medical monitors as opposed to conventional compu-ter monitors. If such studies could be implemented on a larger scale to convince medical practitioners as well as the legal institutions, it is very likely that a good lossy compression may be accepted for radiologic images in teleradiology. Even at the current time, many busy radiologists view their patient images at their own computer in their offices, albeit with the lower resolution and image quality via Web-based tools such as MagicView used in Siemens systems.

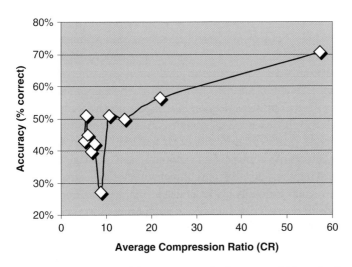

Fig. 3.3. The accuracy of diagnosis on medical images at different levels of lossy compression

A study on the image characteristics and clinical considerations for radiologic image compression in [10] claims that the two main components of interest to maintain higher image quality in radiologic image compression are sharp edges and general textures. It recommends that many compression methods are suitable for clinical implementation with some clinical guidance and technical modifications. Many lossless techniques can be readily converted to lossy techniques by incorporating some subsampling (e.g., reducing the number of images, frames, or data points stored), discrete analysis, or quantization. Current popular lossy (irreversible) methods for medical images, as discussed in [19], include the 2D discrete cosine transform (DCT), full-frame DCT, lapped orthogonal transform, subband coding, vector quantization, quadtrees, and adaptive predictive coding schemes.

Many image preprocessing techniques incorporate lossy methods in order to reduce the image noise, which is what was done in a controlled manner in the abovementioned study, as shown in Fig. 3.3. With the advances in medical image processing and successful attempts at automated and semiautomated diagnosis (e.g., [11]), it is realized that medical experts are now becoming more savvy in using such technology and are even showing preference for it. ROI, structure, disease modeling, and highlighting are becoming more sought after in analyzing radiologic images. Models often take up less storage than actual raw images that may contain an amount of unnecessary information. Studies such as that reported in [12] indicate that 2D and 3D models can be effective in producing a good lossy compression performance, in addition to visualizing the structures of interest. It is also shown that when designed well, the models may even be stored in the native image format (in this case, DICOM) and then further compressed using conventional algorithms or even the de facto archiving compression in the PACS environment.

3.5
Future Directions

Recently, there have been a number of studies into remote diagnosis, not just via remote workstations, but even via a personal digital assistant [6] and smartphones through the use of mobile agents. Images to be used will need to be compressed significantly for such devices. As compression generally reduces image complexity, it also aids in improving the algorithm and implementation efficiency of both image processing and regular functionality (e.g., displaying, storing, and editing) tasks in those devices with restricted resources and computing power.

In addition, many powerful automatic algorithms to support image processing, including artificial neural networks (ANN), genetic algorithms, particle swarm optimization, wavelets (including directional wavelets), fractals, etc., can also contribute to better compression through their abilities in prediction, approximation, and optimal selection of important information or features in images. In the case of ANN, for instance, various ANN architectures were analyzed in [8], and it has been shown that ANN can contribute to almost every step of the image-processing chain, including image reconstruction, restoration, enhancement, feature extraction, segmentation, object recognition, image understanding, optimization, and, of course, compression. Even when it is not the main objective, lossy compression does get implemented at most of the stages mentioned in one or more indirect ways. Consequently, as lossy techniques become more widespread in medical applications, it is expected that legal and diagnostic considerations will be made to accommodate such compression, especially with respect to the archiving of at least part of the large repository of historic patient records in medical institutions.

3.6
Conclusion

In this chapter, it is seen that with the need to reduce storage requirements, transmission cost, and implementation of modern image-processing techniques, radiologic image compression is inevitable. From the trends observed, in addition to the current widespread use of lossless compression, there will be an increasing acceptance in the use of lossy techniques for these images. These will be applicable to images in two dimensions, three dimensions, or even higher dimensions (inclusive of temporal or frequency information added to the images). It has also been shown that studies conducted have indicated that the diagnostic quality of radiologic images may even be improved through the use of controlled lossy compression. The choice of compression techniques in many institutions is currently limited by the proprietary system of the imaging equipment manufacturers and the PACS, but it is believed that with the ever-increasing number and type of high-performance compression algorithms available on various platforms, a much larger variety of techniques will be made available for use in teleradiology.

Summary

- Compression is necessary for storage and transmission of the large numbers of radiologic images in hospitals.
- Many lossless and lossy compression algorithms are available.
- Good lossy compression has statistically no observable difference from lossless compression.

- A study has shown that lossy compression may be beneficial for diagnosis.
- Modeling provides better visualization and good lossy compression.
- A future trend is to use more compression, likely lossy compression, in image-processing algorithms and for remote diagnosis.
- Legal considerations for accepting lossy compression must be addressed.

References

1. Bilgin A, Zweig G, Marcellin MW (1998) Efficient lossless coding of medical image volumes using reversible integer wavelet transforms. In: Proceedings of data compression conference. IEEE Computer Society Press Los Alamitos, CA , USA. pp 428–437
2. Chen F, Sahni S, Vemuri BC (1999) Efficient algorithms for lossless compression of 2D/3D images. VISUAL'99. Lecture Notes in Computer Science, vol 1614. Springer, Heidelberg, pp 681–688
3. Choong MK (2004) Digitisation, lossy compression and visualisation in cost-effective telehealth environment. Master of Engineering Science thesis, Multimedia University, Melaka, Malaysia
4. Choong M-K, Logeswaran R, Bister M (2006) Improving diagnostic quality of MR images through controlled lossy compression using SPIHT. J Med Sys 30(3):139–143
5. Choong M-K, Logeswaran R, Bister M (2007) Cost-effective handling of digital medical images in the telemedicine environment. Intl J Med Inform 76(9):646–654
6. Chung S-H, Logeswaran R (2005) Mobile agents in mobile telemedicine—replication agent and snapshot agent approach to overcome wireless bandwidth limitation. Multimedia Cyberscape J 3(4):41–45
7. Clunie DA (2002) NEMA DICOM status update—DICOM compression 2002. SPIE: medical imaging 2002. International Society of Optical Engineering, San Diego
8. Egmont-Petersen M, de Ridder D Handels H (2002) Image processing with neural networks—a review. Pattern Recognit 35:2279–2301
9. Lemke HU, Osteaux M (eds) (1993) Picture archiving and communication systems and digital radiology. Eur J Radiol 17(1):1–2
10. Lo S-C, Kim M-B, Li H, Krasner BH, Freedman MT, Mun SK (1994) Radiological image compression: image characteristics and clinical considerations. Proc SPIE 2164:276–281
11. Logeswaran R (2007) A computer-aided multi-disease diagnostic system using MRCP. J Digit Imaging. doi:10.1007/s10278-007-9029-4
12. Logeswaran R, Eswaran C (2006) Model-based compression for 3D medical images stored in the DICOM format. J Med Sys 30(2):133–138
13. Marcelo A, Fontelo P, Farolan M, Cualing H (2000) Effect of image compression on telepathology: a randomized clinical trial. Arch Pathol Lab Med 124(11):1653–1656
14. NEMA (1996) Digital imaging and communications in medicine (DICOM). National Electrical Manufacturers' Association, Rosslyn, PS 3.1-1996–3.13-1996
15. Perlmutter SM, Cosman PC, Gray RM et al (1997) Image quality in lossy compressed digital mammograms. Signal Process 59(2):189–210
16. Said A, Pearlman WA (1996) A new, fast, and efficient image codec based on set partitioning in hierarchical trees. IEEE Trans Circuits Syst Video Technol 6(3):243–250

17. Seward J. Bzip2. http://www.bzip.org/
18. Sharpiro JM (1993) Embedded image coding using zerotrees of wavelet coefficients. IEEE Trans Signal Process 41(12):3445–3462
19. Wong S, Zaremba L, Gooden D, Huang HK (1996) Radiologic image compression—a review. Proc IEEE 83(2):194–219
20. Wu X, Menon N (1996) CALIC—a context based adaptive lossless image codec. In: Proceedings of international conference on acoustics, speech, and signal processing. IEEE Signal Processing Society Press ISBN: 0780331923 pp 1890–1893

4

DICOM Image Secure Communication with Internet Protocols

Jianguo Zhang

Abstract Teleradiology systems are developed for the exchange of medical imaging data. In teleradiology, DICOM communication service is used to deliver image data from a requester site to an expert site or vice versa. At present, two methods provide secure communication channels with TCP/IP-based DICOM image communication protocols: IPSec and SSL/TLS. DICOM specifies a Web-based service called WADO for accessing and presenting images, medical imaging reports, etc. from HTML pages or XML documents. An electronic health-care record system needs to be developed as an information-exchanging platform for regional coordinated health-care services and security measures need to be taken to ensure data privacy, authentication, and integrity.

4.1
Introduction

Data privacy, authenticity, and integrity are three critical issues for the development of teleradiology systems involved in the exchange of medical imaging data. Three organizations have issued guidelines, mandates, and standards for the secure transmission of medical images and data. First, in 1994, the American College of Radiology issued standards for teleradiology, which define guidelines for both physicians and nonphysician personnel and address equipment specifications, liability, and licensing and credentialing of staff [1, 2, 16, 17]. Second, the Health Insurance Portability and Accountability Act Public Law 104-191, which was adopted in 1996 as an amendment to the Internal Revenue Service Code of 1986, mandates protection of patient privacy and restricts communication of "protected" medical information [3, 4]. Third, Part 15 of the digital imaging and communication in medicine (DICOM) standard specifies technical requirements for software applications used for the exchange of sensitive patient data [18].

Privacy refers to denying access to information by unauthorized individuals. Authenticity refers to validating the source of a message and ensuring that it was

Sending Site   Receiving Site

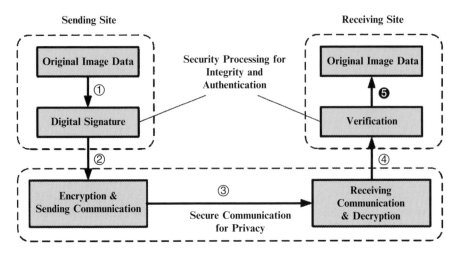

Fig. 4.1. Data flow of medical image secure communication from one site to another through the public Internet

transmitted by a properly identified sender. Integrity refers to the assurance that the data were not modified accidentally or deliberately in transit and by replacement, insertion, or deletion. Figure 4.1 depicts secure image delivery from one site to another through a wide-area network (WAN). There are two processing steps that help to secure the content of delivered images. First, to ensure the integrity and authenticity of the transmitted data, the digest (or hash computing on data) and digital signature, as well as decoding signature and comparing digest, on the images before and after transferring are performed at both the transmitting and the receiving sites [30]. Second, to protect privacy, images are transmitted through secure communication channels.

There are already many publications discussing the technical methods and algorithms of the first of these two security measures [22, 23, 30]. In this chapter, we will focus on the secure communication of medical images.

4.2
Image Communication Modes in Teleradiology

In teleradiology, there are many service models that use different image transmission data flows to deliver image data from a requester site to an expert site. These models include simple, complicated [13], expert-model [26], and central-mode [28] teleradiology. Alternatively, image delivery in teleradiology operates in either "push" or "pull" modes. In push mode, the image data are sent to the expert site or expert center from the requester site directly using the point-to-point (simple and complicated teleradiology) and the many-to-point (expert-model teleradiology) models. In these models, data transmission can be completed using the DICOM storage (C-Store) communication service. The sender side is called C-Store service class user (SCU), and the receiver side is called C-Store service class provider (SCP). If the communication protocol of pull mode uses DICOM, there will be at least two DICOM communication services involved in this mode. One is the DICOM storage service (C-Store SCU/SCP), which is used to send the image data from requester sites to the data center or repository or from the data center or repository to an expert site. The second service is the DICOM query/retrieval service, which is used to query and locate patient image data (C-Find SCU/SCP) and then to retrieve or pull the data (C-Move SCU/SCP and C-Store SCU/SCP).

Regardless of the image delivery mode used, there are presently two methods to provide secure communication channels with transmission control protocol (TCP)/Internet protocol (IP) based DICOM image communication protocols: IP security (IPSec) and secure socket layer (SSL)/transport-layer security (TLS). In the next section, we will discuss the implementation of the TCP/IP version 6 (IPv6)/IP version 4 (IPv4) enabled DICOM communication libraries and application software [29].

4.3
TCP/IPv6/IPv4 Communication Protocols and DICOM Communication Software

4.3.1
Basic Architecture of TCP/IP

Most of today's Internet uses IPv4, which is now nearly 20 years old. IPv4 has been remarkably resilient in spite of its age, but specific problems have now emerged. Most importantly, there is a growing shortage of IPv4 addresses, which are needed by all new machines added to the Internet. Most network applications and protocols (client/server, Web, hypertext transfer protocol, HTTP, DICOM, etc.) used in the Internet or intranet have been developed on the basis of TCP/IPv4, which is partitioned into three layers according to the International Standards Organization open systems interconnection (OSI) definition [15]: the application, transport, and IP layers. Owing to the oversubscription of Internet addresses and the availability of networks with greater bandwidth, TCP/IPv4 has been affected by certain problems, specifically, (1) a shortage of addresses, (2) security is not integrated and IPSec is an add-on, (3) problems of multicasting, (4) complicated headers,

(5) fragmentation/retransmission problems, (6) poor quality of service, (7) inability to handle large frames, and (8) limited autoconfiguration support (needed by dynamic host configuration protocol).

IPv6 is a new version of IP that is designed to be an evolutionary derivative of IPv4 [14]. IPv6 is designed to run well on high-performance networks (e.g., gigabit Ethernet, OC-12, ATM, etc.) and at the same time still be efficient for low-bandwidth networks (e.g., wireless). In addition, it provides a platform for higher-speed Internet functionality. IPv6 was designed to solve many of the problems of the current version of IPv4, specifically, address depletion, security, autoconfiguration, extendability, etc. IPv6 includes many associated protocols such as IPSec, Internet control message protocol for IPv6 (ICMPv6), etc. IPv6 has some special features such as (1) larger address space, (2) aggregation-based address hierarchy and efficient backbone routing, (3) efficient and extensible IP datagram such as no fragmentation by routers, 64-bit field alignment, and simple basic header, (4) autoconfiguration, (5) security, and (6) IP renumbering as part of the protocol. Figure 4.2 shows the architecture of TCP/IPv4 and TCP/IPv6, from which we see that the major differences between TCP/IPv4 and TCP/IPv6 are in the IP layer. Also, IPSec is integrated into IPv6 as the default security protocol, whereas SSL was adopted to provide

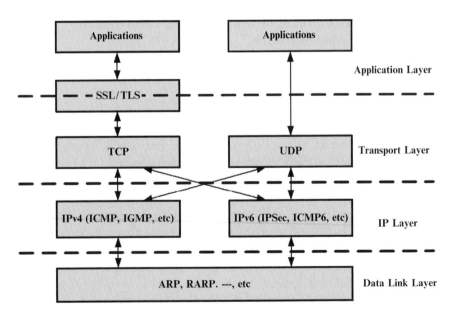

Fig. 4.2. Transmission control protocol (*TCP*)/Internet protocol version 4 (*IPv4*)/Internet protocol version 6 (*IPv6*) family architecture

security channels in the application layer in the IPv4 network environment. By comparison, IPSec was added to IPv4 later on.

4.3.2
DICOM Communication Software

Most medical image communication software employs DICOM communication services to transfer image data between imaging modalities, picture archiving and communication systems (PACS) archiving servers, workstations, and other components, as well as between teleradiology systems and in enterprise PACS environments with WAN interconnections. In DICOM, the OSI basic reference model is used to model the interconnection of medical imaging equipment, as shown in Fig. 4.3. DICOM uses the OSI upper-layer service to separate the exchange of DICOM messages and objects at the application layer from the communication support provided by the lower layers. This OSI upper layer service boundary allows peer application entities to establish associations, transfer messages, and terminate associations. As indicated in Fig. 4.3, the upper-layer protocol augmenting TCP/IP is now adopted by most DICOM communication applications to transfer and deliver DICOM messages or image objects between equipment and devices. As such, the major tasks to

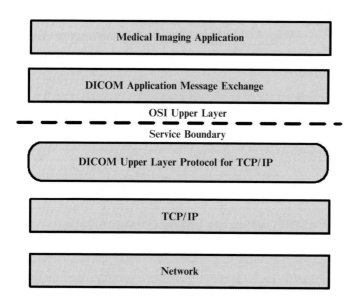

Fig. 4.3. Digital imaging and communication in medicine (*DICOM*) network communication protocols architecture

implement DICOM communication software involve developing application program interface (APIs) and implementing DICOM upper-layer protocols with TCP/IPv4 in various computer platforms.

In order to enable medical image transmission through high-speed broadband networks with IPv6, the DICOM upper-layer protocol with TCP/IPv6 needs to be developed and made compatible with IPv4. There are toolkits that provide open-source reference implementation of the DICOM standard, such as central test node (CTN) DICOM toolkit, which was developed by the Mallinckrodt Institute of Radiology in St. Louis (USA) [20], and the OFFIS DICOM toolkit DCMTK, which was developed in Oldenburg (Germany) [5]. (These two open-source software programs have implemented most of the APIs of the DICOM upper-layer protocol for TCP/IPv4 for different operating systems) (UNIX/Windows/Linux).)

In the following sections, we present an approach to select the CTN DICOM toolkit to implement the DICOM upper layer for TCP/IPv6. This approach has served as a test bed for cross-vendor testing of DICOM communication services [20]. The implementation was straightforward: For software, it only needs to replace the original TCP/IPv4 socket functions with requests for comments standard TCP/IPv6/v4-compatible socket functions, provided by each operating system; recompile the software; and link it to the DICOM application services. For each operating environment, the IPv6 stack software needs to be installed and used to perform some reconfigurations, such as assigning IP addresses and configuring the tunnel in the specific operation system, such as Windows XP, Linux (e.g., Red Hat version 3.0 and above), and Solaris (version 7.0 and above), which already support IPv6. As a result, we have developed IPv6/IPv4-enabled DICOM communication services and applications:

- DICOM C-Store SCU and SCP
- DICOM C-Find SCU and SCP
- DICOM C-Move SCU and SCP
- DICOM QUERY/RETRIEVE SCU and SCP

4.4
Implementation of DICOM Secure Image Communication Protocols

DICOM standard Part 15 (PS 3.15-2007) provides a standardized method for ensuring secure communication and digital signature verification. It specifies technical means (selection of security standards, algorithms, and parameters) for application entities involved in exchanging information to implement security policies. The implementation of the DICOM Part 15 secure transport connection profiles for DICOM image security transmission utilizes the framework and negotiation mechanism specified by TLS version 1.0, which is derived from SSL version 3.0. The secure communication of IPv6-enabled DICOM image transmission utilizes IPsec, which is now mostly used in virtual private network (VPN) applications and will be widely used in high-speed broadband networks. In this section, we first provide the software implementations of IPv6/IPv4 secure DICOM communication with IPsec supported and then discuss the SSL/TLS-based DICOM secure communication. In the next section, we describe experiments and compare the efficiencies of both secure DICOM communication methods, namely, IPSec-based and SSL/TLS-based, with different modality DICOM images, secure algorithms, and computer platforms [29].

4.4.1
DICOM Communication with IPSec-Based Security Supported

Figure 4.2 demonstrates that IPSec is a member of the IPv6 family. It provides security to the IP and the upper-layer protocols. IPSec is composed of two protocols: the authentication header (AH) and the encapsulating security payload (ESP) protocols. AH is used to ensure the authentication and integrity of the message, while ESP is used to ensure confidentiality. The AH protocol uses hash message authentication codes to protect integrity. Many algorithms can be used in AH, such as secure hash algorithm, Message Digest-5, etc. [10]. The ESP protocol uses the standard symmetric encryption algorithms to protect confidentiality, such as triple data encryption standard, advanced encryption standard, 448-bit Blowfish encryption algorithm, etc. [10].

Figure 4.4 shows the data flow of the service pairs of the IPv6/IPv4 DICOM storage SCU and SCP with IPsec-supported security. The DICOM SCU and SCP have their own certificates, which are created by the same certificate authority. There are three steps in IPsec communication. The first is Internet key exchange (IKE) protocol association. In this step, the Internet security association and key management protocol demons running in both SCU and SCP sites negotiate the IKE parameters and exchange certificates, which are used for IPSec association. In the second step, the SCU and SCP entities establish DICOM associations, which include the IPSec association. In this step, both sites negotiate IPSec parameters and create session keys, which are used for secure communication of DICOM data. The third step is transferring the DICOM data on the secure channel.

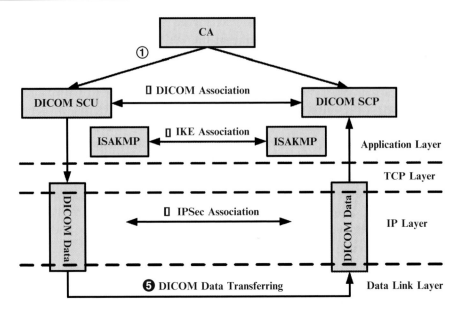

Fig. 4.4. The data flow of TCP/IPv6-based DICOM C-Store communication with Internet protocol security (*IPSec*) security supported. First, the certificate authority (*CA*) assigns the X.509 certificate to service class user (*SCU*) and service class provider (*SCP*) sites, respectively, prior to the testing, and the Internet security association and key management protocol (*ISAKMP*) demons running in both SCU and SCP sites create the Internet key exchange (*IKE*) association, negotiate the IKE parameters, and exchange certificates that are used for IPSec association. Second, the SCU and SCP entities establish DICOM association including IPSec association, and both sites negotiate IPSec parameters and create a session key. Third, the SCU transfers the DICOM data to the SCP through IPSec-based secure channels

IPSec works in two modes: tunnel and transport modes. In tunnel mode the entire IP datagram is encapsulated by a new datagram that includes the outer IP header, IP header, and IP payload, while in transport mode it only handles the payload (upper-layer data) by inserting AHs, ESP headers, or both. Since the tunnel mode needs to configure routing in network communications and transmission performance, it would be affected by the network hardware selected and it does not truly represent IPsec performance. For this reason, we only evaluated the transport mode.

Since the secure operation is in the IP layer, IPSec has no effect on DICOM communication entities, which work in the application layer. To test the performance of DICOM communication with IPSec-supported security, we need to set up security associations (SA) for peer entities to establish the secure channel. During the setup process, we create certificates for both peers and set SA-associated parameters.

4.4.2
DICOM Image Communication with SSL/TLS-Based Security Supported

The SSL was originally developed by Netscape Communications to allow secured access of a browser to a Web server and has since become the accepted standard for Web security [21]. It provides secure communication channels between clients and servers by allowing mutual authentication, which uses digital signatures for integrity and encryption for privacy. The protocol was designed to support multiple choices of specific algorithms used for cryptography, digests, and signatures. SSL 3.0 is the basis for the TLS protocol, which is still being developed by the Internet Engineering Task Force [6, 7]. The SSL protocol uses both public-key and symmetric-key encryptions. Symmetric-key encryption is much faster than public-key encryption, but public-key encryption provides better authentication techniques.

SSL consists of two protocols: the handshake and the SSL record protocols. The handshake protocol defines how the peer entities exchange associated information, such as SSL version, ciphers, and authentication certificates. The SSL record protocol defines the format of the SSL record or message, in which all of the SSL-associated messages or application data should be transferred. The SSL connection is executed in two phases: handshake and data transfer.

The data flow of the DICOM storage SCU and SCP entities with SSL/TLS-supported security is shown in Fig. 4.5. SSL/TLS works between the TCP layer and the application layer. Most implementations of the SSL (version 3.0)/TLS communication library simulate the style of the Berkeley socket APIs [11]. In the implementation of DICOM secure image communication with the SSL/TLS-supported security, the TCP APIs (socket functions) were replaced with DICOM secure image by using the open SSL toolkit of the SSL (version 3.0)/TLS communication library in the DICOM CTN library software; the CTN library was recompiled and the application was linked to the SSL/TLS-based DICOM secure communication library.

4.5
Performance Evaluation of DICOM Image Secure Communication Protocols

The transmission performance of TCP/IP for medical image communication with IPsec- or SSL/TLS-supported security depends on various parameters, including transmission protocol, protocol data unit (PDU) size, security algorithm, and computer operating system. It also depends on the types of images being transmitted. We designed a set of image transmission experiments by permuting these

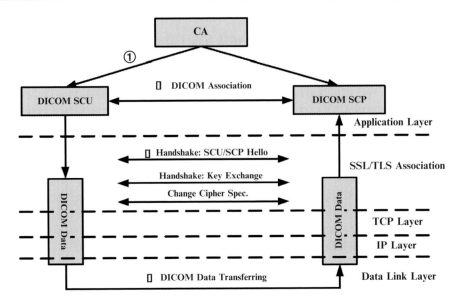

Fig. 4.5. The data flow of DICOM C-Store communication through secure socket layer(*SSL*)/ transport-layer security (*TLS*) secure channels: First, the CA assigns the X.509 certificates to SCU and SCP sites, respectively, prior to testing. Second, SCU and SCP establish DICOM associations, which execute SSL handshakes. Third, the DICOM SCU transforms the DICOM data into an SSL record format and sends it to the SCP through SSL secure channels; the DICOM SCP performs the reverse process and gets the original DICOM data

parameters, in order to evaluate DICOM image communication performance under various conditions. We also compared the measured results.

We used the DICOM C-STORE DICOM message service element as an example to evaluate the DICOM transmission performance of computed tomography (CT), magnetic resonance (MR), computed radiography (CR), and multiframe ultrasound images in different security environments [29]. We used two computers; one worked as the DICOM C-STORE SCU for sending images and the other served as the DICOM C-STORE SCP for receiving images. We performed three exhaustive experiments to evaluate secured DICOM communication protocols under various conditions and parameters, such as TCP/IP (IPv6 and IPv4), security configurations (IPSec and SSL/TLS), algorithms, and PDU sizes. We have following conclusions [29]:

- There are some overheads (transmission rates were slightly decreased) in using IPv6 DICOM image communication compared with IPv4, since more advanced features are achieved in IPv6 and more protocols are performed on the transmitted data.

- All encryption algorithms used in IPsec- and SSL/TLS-based securities slow down transmission performance of CR and multiframe ultrasound (or digital subtraction angiography) images compared with that of CT and MR images in TCP/IPv6/IPv4 networking. All encryption algorithms used in IPsec- and SSL/TLS-based securities reduce the rates of transmission of CR, multiframe ultrasound, and digital subtraction angiography images more than they reduce the rates for CT and MR images in TCP/Ipv6/Ipv4 networks.
- Transmission of DICOM images can occur faster over TCP/IPv4 networks than over TCP/IPv6 networks if IPsec-based security is not enabled. When IPsec-based security is enabled, the integration of IPv6 and IPSec is better than that of IPv4 with IPsec.
- Transmission rates for DICOM images with different SSL/TLS security algorithms over TCP/IPv4 networks in Linux and Windows are faster than those with the same security settings but cross-platforms such as SCU (Linux) to SCP (Windows).

There is a trade-off in choosing IPsec-based implementation instead of SSL/TLS-based security implementation of IPv6/IPv4. If WAN networks use IPv6 as the only transmission protocol in the next generation of high-performance broadband networks, then the ideal choice is IPsec-based security. This is because IPv6 and IPsec are implemented in the IP layer and no changes in application software would be needed. However, the operating systems would have to be reconfigured to enable the IPv6 to be integrated with IPsec security. If the networks use IPv4 or a combination of IPv6 and IPv4, it is better to use SSL/TLS security by modifying the TCP/IP APIs of the application software. This is because the integration of IPv4 with IPsec is not as good as with IPsec alone. Alternatively, it may be better to find a VPN product. However, in the latter case, there are certain limitations in network deployment.

The Linux platform achieves better performance and has more security algorithms implemented than the Windows (XP) platform in most studies of IPv6- and IPv4-based DICOM image communication. In teleradiology and enterprise PACS applications, the Linux operating system may be a better choice as the peer security gateway for both IPsec- and SSL/TLS-based secure DICOM communications crosses public networks. Otherwise, the Windows platform could be better if the speed of data communication is the most important consideration. Of note, the combination of Linux and Windows platforms, such as Linux with SCU and Windows with SCP in secured DICOM communications, did not have as good transmission performance as did either platform operating separately. Since most Linux operating systems are derived from UNIX operating systems, most of the conclusions reported in the present study may be applicable to UNIX platforms as well.

4.6
DICOM Image Secure Communication in Web Applications

Medical research, education, teleradiology, and telemedicine may require access to hospital image archiving servers or repositories through a local-area network or a WAN, for the purposes of medical research, education, and even telemedicine. Cost-effective image delivery and display are needed in most networked hospitals. Web-based medical image systems are the most effective solution for these purposes because they employ the HTTP communication protocol and browsers, which are more universal and convenient than DICOM communication protocols [27]. Also, Part 18 of the DICOM standard specifies a Web-based service called Web access DICOM persistent object (WADO) for accessing and presenting DICOM persistent objects (e.g., images and medical imaging reports) [19]. The WADO is intended for distribution of results and images to health-care professionals. It provides a simple mechanism for accessing a DICOM persistent object from HTML pages or XML documents using HTTP/HTTP over SSL (HTTPS) and DICOM unique identifiers. Data may be retrieved either in a presentation-ready form as specified by the requester, e.g., Joint Photographic Experts Group format or Graphics Interchange Format, or in a DICOM native format.

In Web-based image-distribution applications, the image transmission usually occurs through the HTTP. For secure image transferring through a WAN, the image application clients and servers should enable the HTTPS for data transfer. Presently, we define HTTP and HTTPS and explain how they work and how to use them.

HTTP is an application-level protocol for distributed, collaborative, hyper-media information systems, which goes over TCP/IP connections and uses request/response operation models to transfer data [12]. A client sends a request to the server in the form of a request method, URI, and protocol version, followed by a MIME-like message containing request modifiers, client information, and possible body content over a connection with a server. The server responds with a status line, including the message's protocol version and a success or error code, followed by a MIME-like message containing server information, entity meta-information, and possible entity-body content. HTTPS is a Web protocol originally developed by Netscape (now a subsidiary of America Online) [24], and it can encrypt and decrypt user page requests as well as the pages that are returned by the Web server. HTTPS is really just the use of SSL as a sublayer under its regular HTTP application layer. It uses a certificate and a public key to encrypt data to be transferred over the Internet.

Now, most popular Web servers and client products, such as Microsoft Internet Information Server, Internet Explorer browser, and Apache/Tomcat Web servers support HTTPS, and it is fairly straightforward to use HTTPS to securely transfer image data in Web applications, if one follows the instructions for Web products provided by vendors to configure Web servers and clients.

4.7
Future Directions and Applications of DICOM Image Secure Communication

Images, diagnostic reports, and evidence documents derived from the processing of images represent important components of a patient's medical record. A number of health-care delivery professionals (e.g., referring physicians, radiologists, surgeons, oncologists) would benefit from a coordinated method for locating and accessing relevant imaging information. The creation and subsequent usage of these documents may span several health-care delivery organizations through a WAN and may be performed separately over different time periods. Thus, the electronic health-care record system (EHRS) needs to be rapidly developed as an information-exchange platform for regional coordinated health-care services, and many security measures need to be applied to ensure data privacy, authentication, and integrity. The EHRS is a secure, real-time, point-of-care, patient-centric information resource for health-care providers. Many countries and regional districts, such as the National Programme for IT in the UK and the Healthcare Infoway project in Canada, have set long-term goals to build an EHRS, and most of the EHRS is usually built on the basis of the integration of different information systems with different information models and platforms.

One of key integration problems in of the development of an EHRS is the inability to share and exchange patient records among various hospitals and health-care providers. To solve this integration problem, Integrating Healthcare Enterprise (IHE) [25] has defined an integration profile called cross-enterprise document sharing (XDS) to regulate the sharing of data contained in medical records [9]. The XDS for images (XDS-I) profile [8], depending on the IHE information technology infrastructure (ITI) XDS profile, extends and specializes XDS to support imaging "documents," specifically including sets of DICOM instances (including images, evidence documents, presentation states, and diagnostic imaging reports provided in a ready-for-display format). Also, some security integration profiles, e.g., IHE IT technical framework: audit trial and node authentication (ATNA), enterprise user authentication (EUA), and ITI technical framework supplement digital signature [8, 9], have been developed to provide technical guidance in making the EHRS more secure.

Since most transactions from imaging document source actors to consumer actors are still based on DICOM, the topics discussed in this chapter are still very relevant in the development of an EHRS. The implementation of DICOM image secure communication in an EHRS is still a challenging issue in cross-vendor health-care information systems. Another challenge is how to integrate different security components, such as ATNA, EUA, single sign-on, and digital signature, to provide complete and seamless security solutions for enterprise and cross-enterprise health-care services.

Summary

- Teleradiology systems are developed for the exchange of medical imaging data.
- In teleradiology, the DICOM communication service is used to deliver image data from a requester site to an expert site or vice versa.
- At present, two methods provide secure communication channels with TCP/IP-based DICOM image communication protocols: IPSec and SSL/TLS.
- DICOM specifies a Web-based service called WADO for accessing and presenting images, medical imaging reports, etc. from HTML pages or XML documents.
- An electronic health-care record system needs to be developed as an information-exchange platform for regional coordinated health-care services and security measures need to be taken to ensure data privacy, authentication, and integrity.

References

1. Berger SB, Cepelewicz BB (1996) Medical–legal issues in teleradiology. Am J Roentgenol 166:505–502
2. Berlin L (1998) Malpractice issue in radiology–teleradiology. Am J Roentgenol 170:1417–1422
3. HIPAA. http://www.rx2000.org/KnowledgeCenter/hipaa/hipfaq.htm. Last Accessed date 02 May 2008
4. HIPAA, US Department of Health and Human Services. http://aspe.os.dhhs.gov/admnsimp
5. http://dicom.offis.de/dcmtk.php.en
6. http://www.ietf.org/
7. http://www.ihe.net/Technical_Framework/upload/ihe_RAD_TF_Suppl_XDSI_TI_2005-08-15.pdf
8. http://www.ihe.net/Technical_Framework/upload/IHE_ITI_TF-Supplement_Digital_Signature-TI_2005-08-15.pdf
9. http://www.ihe.net/Technical_Framework/upload/IHE_ITI_TF_2.0_vol1_FT_2005-08-15.pdf
10. http://www.ipsec-howto.org/
11. http://www.openssl.org/

12. http://www.w3.org/ Protocols/rfc2068

13. Huang HK (1996) Teleradiology technologies and some service models. Comput Med Imaging Graph 20:59–68

14. Huitema C (1999) IPV6 the new Internet protocol. Prentice-Hall, Upper Saddle River,

15. International Organization for Standardization. http://www.iso.org

16. James AE Jr, James E III, Johnson B, James J (1993) Legal considerations of medical of medical imaging. Leg Med 87–113

17. Kamp GH (1996) Medical–legal issues in teleradiology: a commentary. Am J Roentgenol 166:511–512

18. NEMA (2007) Digital imaging and communications in medicine (DICOM). Part 15: security and system management profiles, PS 3.15-2007. National Electrical Manufacturers Association, Rosslyn. http://medical.nema.org/dicom/2007

19. NEMA (2007) Digital Imaging and Communications in Medicine (DICOM). Part 18: web access to DICOM persistent objects (WADO), PS 3.18-2007. National Electrical Manufactures Association, Rosslyn. http://medical.nema.org/dicom/2007

20. Radiological Society of North America, Mallinckrodt Institute of Radiology. Overview of 1997 RSNA DICOM demonstration. file:/wuerlb/documentation/dicom/dicom.97/ overview.doc

21. Rescorla E (2001) SSL and TLS: designing and building secure systems. Addison-Wesley, Boston

22. Rives R, Shamir A, Adleman L (1978) A method for obtaining digital signatures and public-key cryptosystems. Commun ACM 21(2):120–126

23. Wong STC, Abundo M, Huang HK (1995) Authenticity techniques for PACS images and records. SPIE Med Imaging 2435:68–79

24. http://www.aol.com

25. http://www.ihe.org/

26. Zhang J, Stahl N, Huang HK, Zhou X, Lou SL, Song KS (2000) Real-time teleconsultation with high resolution and large volume medical images for collaborative health care. IEEE Trans Inform Technol Biomed 4:178–186

27. Zhang J, Sun J, Stahl JN (2003) PACS and web based image distribution and display. Comput Med Imaging Graph 27:197–206

28. Zhang J, Sun J, Yang Y et al (2005) Web-based electronic patient records for collaborative medical applications. Comput Med Imaging Graph 29:115–124

29. Zhang J, Yu F, Sun J, Yang Y, Liang C (2007) DICOM image secure communications with Internet protocols IPv6 and IPv4. IEEE Trans Inform Technol Biomed 11(1):70–80

30. Zhou X, Huang HK, Lou SL (2001) Authenticity and integrity of digital mammography images. IEEE Trans Med Imaging 20(8):784–791

5

Radiological Tele-immersion

Zhuming Ai, Bei Jin, and Mary Rasmussen

Abstract It is important to make patient-specific data quickly available and usable to many specialists at different geographical sites. A tele-immersive radiological system has been developed for remote consultation, surgical preplanning, postoperative evaluation, and education. Tele-immersive devices include personal augmented reality immersive system, configurable wall, physician's personal virtual reality display, ImmersaDesk, volume rendering, cluster-based visualization of large-scale volumetric data, tele-immersive collaboration, and system implementation.

5.1
Introduction

Since the acquisition of high-resolution three-dimensional (3D) patient images has become widespread, medical volumetric data sets (computed tomography, CT, or magnetic resonance imaging, MRI) larger than 100 MB and encompassing more than 250 slices are common. The value of information acquisition is not simply to acquire data at increased precision; it is important to make this patient-specific data quickly available and usable to many specialists at different geographical sites.

Visualization of radiological volumetric data is widely used in medical and biomedical research, diagnoses, training, and education. Efforts have been made to address the problems of how to organize, manage, and present large data sets to specialists at different geographical locations. Hendin et al. [5] have presented methods to provide volume rendering over the Internet. Web-based systems have been developed to provide volume or surface rendering of medical data over networks with low fidelity [17, 18]. However, these cannot adequately handle stereoscopic visualization, huge data sets, and the need for real-time communication between the clinicians. Various restrictions, including interactive latency, viewing orientation, and quality of data representation, exist.

State-of-the-art virtual reality (VR) techniques and high-speed networks have made it possible to create an environment for clinicians geographically distributed to immersively share these massive data sets in real time.[9] Tele-immersion is the integration of audioconferencing and videoconferencing with collaborative VR in the context of data-mining and significant computation. When participants are tele-immersed, they are able to see and interact with each other in a shared environment. Successful demonstrations of tele-immersive biomedical environments have been produced, including the virtual temporal bone [14] and the virtual pelvic floor [12]. A tele-immersive medical educational environment has been created [1]. Advanced network features of the next-generation Internet, such as quality of service, data privacy, and security, will permit tele-immersive environments derived from models of patient data. This may ultimately have widespread impact on daily practice of surgical specialties.

We have developed a networked collaborative system for tele-immersive consultation, surgical preplanning, postoperative evaluation, and education. A method for instantaneously importing medical volumetric data into tele-immersive environments has been developed.

5.2
Tele-immersive Devices

Tele-immersion enables users in different locations to collaborate in a shared, virtual, or simulated environment, as if they are in the same room. It is the ultimate synthesis of networking and media technologies to enhance collaborative environments. Tele-immersive applications combine audio, avatars (representations of participants), virtual worlds, computation, and teleconferencing into an integrated networked system [8]. With use of advanced networks and advanced visualization techniques, a cutting-edge tele-immersive radiology system has been created. This system is a networked tele-immersive collaborative system for surgical preplanning, consultation, postoperative evaluation, and education.

Four different VR systems are used in this networked tele-immersive radiological environment: a personal augmented reality immersive system (PARIS™), a configurable wall (C-Wall), an ImmersaDesk™, and a physician's personal VR display (Fig. 5.1). Physicians in different locations can work together in this tele-immersive environment.

5.2.1
Personal Augmented Reality Immersive System

The PARIS used in this study (Fig. 5.2) is an augmented reality device with a $5' \times 4'$ screen that uses a digital light processing (DLP) projector to display 3D stereo images with a $1,400 \times 1,050$ pixel resolution. A half-silvered mirror

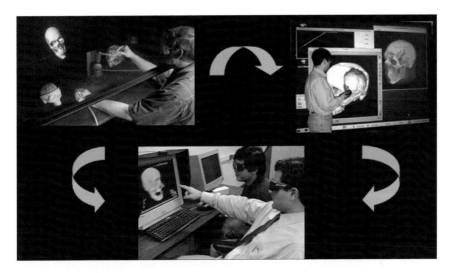

Fig. 5.1. Tele-immersive virtual reality (VR) environment

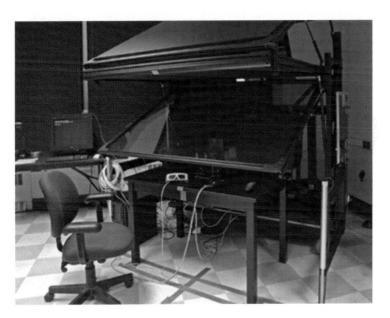

Fig. 5.2. The personal augmented reality immersive system (PARIS)

mounted at an angle in front of the viewer prevents the computer-generated image from being blocked by the user's hands. This not only provides augmented reality but also avoids an important stereo vision depth perception conflict.

A tracking system with two sensors has been installed on the PARIS. One of the sensors is mounted on a pair of liquid crystal display shutter glasses to track the movement of the viewer's head. The other is mounted inside a 3D interactive device, Wanda, to track the movement of the user's hand. The system can generate stereo images from the viewer's perspective and let the user interact with the data directly in three dimensions. A SensAble Technologies PHANTOM® desktop haptic device [6] is mounted on a desk in the PARIS to provide a sense of touch. This system combines VR, augmented reality, and haptic reality.

A Linux personal computer (PC) is used to drive the PARIS. The PC controls two display devices at the same time: one is the projector on the PARIS and the other is an ordinary monitor attached to the PARIS. This second monitor is used to show the graphical user interface (GUI). With this dual-display configuration, we can separate the two-dimensional (2D) user interface (such as menus, buttons, dialogs, etc.) from the 3D working environment to avoid the complex, and often less effective, 3D user interface programming. The separation of the user interface and the volumetric data visualization working space allows much easier and smoother access to different functions of the application. This second monitor is configured as an independent X Window display. A touch panel screen is also an option as a device for the GUI on the PARIS.

5.2.2
C-Wall

A C-Wall is a tele-immersive display optimized for a conference room or small auditorium. There are many consultation contexts that work best with face-to-face communication, and the C-Wall brings to this environment superior interactive visual display of medical data and the ability to interact over networks with collaborators in remote locations. The C-Wall utilizes two projectors and passive polarization to support stereo.

We have constructed a single-screen, passive stereo C-Wall based on low-cost components (Fig. 5.3). A dual-channel graphics card (NVIDIA Quadro4 980 XGL) is used on a PC to drive the projectors. Two identical DLP projectors (InFocus LP530 with 1024 × 768 pixel resolution) are used to achieve polarized stereo, one for each eye's view. The stereo display uses circular polarizing filters for the two projectors and inexpensive circular polarized glasses. Different polarizing filters are placed in front of each projector lens, and users wear polarizing glasses where each lens only admits the light from the corresponding projector. We chose to use rear projection in our system so that viewers will not block the light from the projectors. A 6′ × 8′ rear-projection screen has been set up. This screen can preserve the polarized light.

In order for the passive stereo to work, the images from the two separate projectors must match up on the screen. The two projectors are stacked on an adjustable

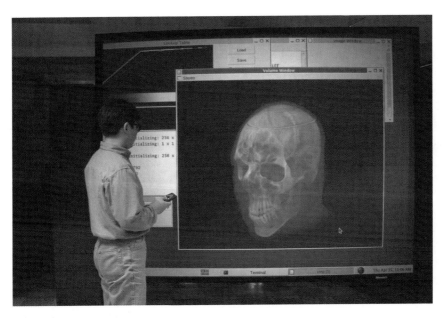

Fig. 5.3. The configurable wall is used to study computed tomography (CT) data

stacker, but not exactly parallel to each other. By tilting one slightly, the two image areas on the screen overlap. The tilted projector's image suffers small keystone distortion in this case, but the error is not significant and is acceptable to users.

5.2.3
Physician's Personal VR Display

The recent development of small Linux PCs and high-performance graphics cards has afforded opportunities to implement applications formerly run on graphics supercomputers. Affordable PC-based VR systems are comparable in performance with expensive graphics supercomputer-based VR systems. Such VR systems can now be accessible to most physicians. The lower cost and smaller size of this system greatly expand the range of uses of VR technology in medicine. With use of PC hardware and other affordable devices, a VR system has been developed which can sit on a physician's desktop or be installed in a conference room.

Because of the need for parallel processing of VR applications, a dual-processor hyperthreading Intel Xeon PC was used in this VR system. NVIDIA Quadro4-based graphics cards perform very well with our application software. Stereo glasses, an emitter, and high-quality CRT monitors were used to generate stereo vision for the desktop configuration (Fig. 5.4).

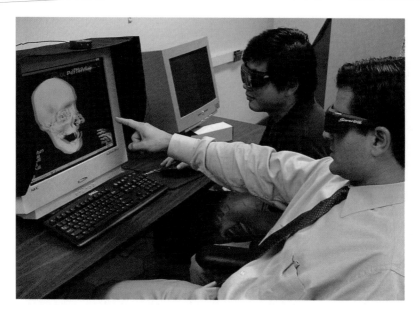

Fig. 5.4. The physician's personal VR display is used to study CT data

5.2.4
ImmersaDesk

The ImmersaDesk [4] is a transportable furniture statement of the cave automatic virtual environment (CAVE™) [3]. This drafting table format of the CAVE provides a large angle of view, stereo vision, and viewer-centered perspective. These are the basic ingredients of any VR display. A 3D mouselike device called the "wand" allows one to interact with and manipulate the virtual environment. Lightweight glasses are used to support stereo vision, and an associated receiver tracks head position, allowing the computer to continually compute the unique perspective view for each eye.

5.3
Volume Rendering

The speed of the volume rendering is a very important issue in radiological tele-immersive applications. In tracked VR devices, the viewer's head is moving constantly, but volume rendering was usually carried out at a much slower rate. The latency between the visual feedback and the movement of the head lowers the quality of the immersive experience. Usually, ten frames per second (fps) refresh rate is considered real time or interactive in computer graphics applications. Classic animation was rendered at 12 fps. In tele-immersive VR applications, a higher frame rate is desired to make the latency unnoticeable and a faster volume rendering algorithm needed to be developed.

The most commonly used volume rendering methods are ray casting [7], 2D texture mapping [15], 3D texture mapping [2], and cluster computing [11]. In this study, a hardware-assisted fast direct volume rendering algorithm has been developed using a commodity PC, Linux operating system, and a NVIDIA graphics card. Three-dimensional texture mapping features available in NVIDIA graphics cards were used to create an application that allows the user to view and interact with CT and MRI data sets. The algorithm supports multiple volumes. Gray-scale volumes of the size of $512 \times 512 \times 256$ can be rendered on a 512×512 window in high quality at a rate of 20 fps.

Three different classification methods (including two preclassification methods and one postclassification method) have been implemented and tested. The classification determines how the value of a voxel is transferred to color or intensity. The first preclassification method makes use of the GL_SHARED_TEXTURE_PALETTE_EXT extension available in NVIDIA's graphics cards. The second preclassification method changes texture before it is sent to graphics hardware. The postclassification method uses the OpenGL shading language. Depending on the ability of the graphics card hardware, a proper classification method was selected automatically to achieve the best performance. We have also implemented a hardware-assisted ray casting volume rendering algorithm. On supported systems, this algorithm can generate better-quality images with a faster rendering speed.

To fully support CT data, 16-bit volume rendering has been implemented. The transfer function editor has been designed to support multiple curves. Users can design multiple curves for the transfer function, and each curve can have a different base color. Gray-scale images with more than 8 bits cannot be displayed without losing information on most display devices. This transfer function editor can assign pseudocolors to a certain range of gray-scale values. This can be used to segment the data and give different tissues different colors. In most classification methods, the transfer function can be changed in real time.

5.4
Visualization of Large-Scale Volumetric Data Using a Computer Cluster

Whole-body CT scans and other radiological techniques have created very large scale volumetric data sets. Because of the restrictions of graphics card texture memory, conventional volume rendering methods can only handle smaller volumes. When one is dealing with large-scale data sets, either the original data are down sampled to lower resolution or only part of the volume is selected for 3D display. Investigators have to trade off between the covered area and the details of the structure. Because of the rapid growth of both the speed and the memory size of high-end PC graphics cards, large-scale volume rendering can be performed on low-cost PC clusters instead of expensive supercomputers. We developed and implemented a volume rendering approach using a high-performance PC cluster server for high-resolution medical volumetric data visualization, to break the limitation on the volume size.

The PC cluster-based volume visualization software program was divided into two parts: a user interface on the VR device and a distributed volume rendering component on the server side. The system allows users to interactively manipulate high-definition large-scale volumetric data in an immersive stereo environment. The distributed volume rendering component performs the actual rendering on the PC cluster.

On the server side, a 20-node PC cluster is used as the renderer for the distributed volume rendering system. The distributed volume rendering component is composed of one master node, one blending node, and several slave nodes, each equipped with an NVIDIA Quadro FX 3000 graphics card (Fig. 5.5). The master node's function is to divide and distribute the volume data to slave nodes. It is the bridge between the client and the cluster. The blending node's task is to collect the subimages from the slave nodes, compositing them into the final full image. The slave rendering nodes mainly perform stereoscopic volume rendering simultaneously on the static subvolumes they keep locally and will update the rendering result whenever the transportation matrix is changed. Sort-last parallel 3D texture volume rendering is the basic algorithm used here to share

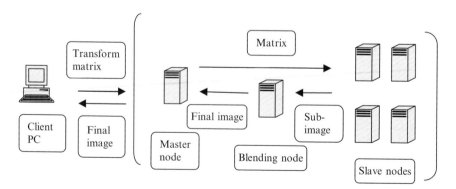

Fig. 5.5. The structure of the cluster-based volume rendering system

the workload among the cluster nodes. We have developed a fast volume rendering algorithm based on 3D texture mapping, and it is used on each slave node.

On the client side, we provided a volume visualization solution that runs locally using modest-performance voxel-based rendering on a commodity PC graphics card. A reduced-resolution version of the large volumetric data set was used to allow interactive manipulation on this computer. We then provide high-performance and large-scale volume rendering by performing the visualization on the cluster and then streaming the result to the client desktop when there is no user interaction.

Because of the size of the data set, the data must be subdivided into smaller bricks and let each node handle one brick. The resulting images from each slave node must be blended together. One of the color-blending algorithms permits layers to be composited in any order while obeying associativity [13]. It permits two four-channel images to compose and yield a new four-channel image. It can be represented as

$$
\begin{aligned}
A_{out} &= A_{fgd} + (1 - A_{fgd}) \times A_{bkg}, \\
C_{0out} &= C_{0fgd} + (1 - A_{fgd}) \times C_{0bkg},
\end{aligned}
$$

where C_{fgd} and C_{bkg} are red, green, or blue components of foreground and background, respectively. A_{fgd} and A_{bkg} are alpha components of foreground and background, respectively. And

$$
\begin{aligned}
C_{0fgd} &= C_{fgd} \times A_{fgd}, \\
C_{0bkg} &= C_{bkg} \times A_{bkg}, \\
C_{0out} &= C_{out} \times A_{out}.
\end{aligned}
$$

This blend function is not directly available in OpenGL or any commodity graphics card. There are two possible ways to implement this blend function. One is to use the existing OpenGL blend function but multiply the original color by its alpha value before it is sent to the OpenGL graphics pipe. The second approach is to use the OpenGL shading language to do this change. Here an OpenGL function is used to take advantage of the graphics card's speed and avoid special hardware requirements. The function glDrawPixel is used to sequentially add images into the frame buffer layer by layer after the rendered images from slave nodes have been sorted from back to front according to the subvolume's position.

The cluster-based volume rendering system has been used to render a volume of the size of 2,000 × 2,800 × 208 voxels. With the accumulated power of the cluster, the system can break the volume size limitation and provide significant accuracy, flexibility, and consistency of rendering. With this system, the user does not have to compromise between the resolution and the data size. The application can display large-scale data in full or interactively zoom into a smaller area to view detailed structure. The cluster-based volume rendering can clarify the full spatial configuration of large-scale radiological data.

5.5
Tele-immersive Collaboration

Collaborative consultation has been implemented in the volume manipulation program (VMP), integrated software that provides volume rendering in a tele-immersive environment. The network component is implemented using the quality of service adaptive networking toolkit (QUANTA) [10], which is a cross-platform adaptive networking toolkit for supporting Optiputer applications over optical networks.

A tele-immersive collaborative VR server has been designed and set up. It has a database to store the shared data, such as CT or MRI data. Collaborators' information is also stored in the database. Client applications can connect to the server to join existing collaborative sessions or open new sessions so that data can be shared among collaborators. Real-time audio communication over the network is implemented among collaborators. Participants are able to speak to each other using the virtual intercom system. It is implemented using the multicasting feature in QUANTA so that it can deliver real-time audio to an unlimited number of collaborators without the concern of bandwidth restrictions. Participants are able to fly through the space using a joystick and interact with the space using buttons on a spatially tracked pointing device, the wand. Each participant can pick, move, and modify any of the objects. As the environment is persistent, participants may exit and reenter the environment at any time.

A network protocol for tele-immersive collaboration has been defined. Currently, it contains the following parts: audio communication, state data sharing, and volumetric data sharing. All the participants in the collaborative session share their viewing angle, transformation matrix, and other application-specific information over the network. Any change made by any one participant is transferred to all other participants. Any changes to the volumetric data are also shared among collaborators.

During collaborative volumetric data manipulation, the changes to the volume are shared in real time among all participants. Only a subvolume that contains the modified data is transferred to other collaborators in order to save bandwidth.

The system is designed to run on different computer systems with different VR devices. The network component makes it possible for people using the application in different environments to share the data and interact with each other in real time.

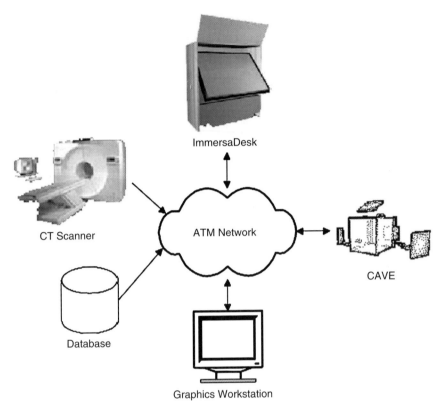

Fig. 5.6. Radiological tele-immersive virtual environment

The radiological tele-immersive environment has been tested on the University of Illinois at Chicago (UIC) campus over the campus network. We tested tele-immersion on several systems at different locations (Fig. 5.6). At the Virtual Reality in Medicine Lab (VRMedLab), a PARIS, an ImmersaDesk, a C-Wall, and a laptop PC were used for the testing. The tele-immersive server is also located at the VRMedLab on a different computer. One and a half miles away on the other side of the campus, another PARIS and a CAVE at the Electronic Visualization Lab were used in the testing. Other nodes can also be added. Computers across the campus are connected over a campus network. The laptop PC was connected to the campus network via Wi-Fi. A CT scan machine in the UIC hospital fed the data into the tele-immersive system.

CT data were pulled directly from the CT scan machine to the tele-immersion server, and then the data were synchronously distributed to all the VR setups. All the clinicians at different VR nodes participated immersively in the same virtual

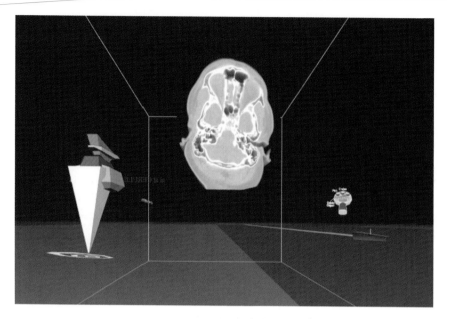

Fig. 5.7. CT data were pulled directly from a CT scan machine and synchronously distributed to all the participants in the tele-immersive virtual environment

environment. When one of them made changes to the model in three dimensions (e.g., moving, rotating, cutting, and windowing), all the other participants saw the changes immediately. With the support of streaming audio communication capability, participants can talk to each other while they are working on the same model. This virtual environment gives the clinicians, who are geographically remote from each other, a virtual conference room, where they can discuss the patient's condition together in real time (Fig. 5.7).

During the test, all computer systems were connected to the server at the same time. When clinicians joined the tele-immersive VR session, the patient's CT data were transferred from the server to each computer and displayed on their display devices. If any one of the users changes the view of the model, all others will see the changes in real time. The PARIS equipped with haptic devices were used to modify the volumetric data collaboratively, and the process can be viewed on all the systems in real time. The tele-immersive session needs to be coordinated in order to prevent users on different systems from manipulating the model at the same time, which may cause some confusion.

The tests were successful and demonstrated that this networked system can be used for remote consultation and evaluation in VR environments as well as in a mobile environment.

5.6
Implementation

The VMP is designed as an integrated volumetric data manipulation program, which has built-in support for tele-immersion. The VMP uses the visualization toolkit [16], a programming interface for creating real-time graphics applications, as its rendering base. The VMP can load common radiology file formats, including digital imaging and communications in medicine (DICOM), and has functionalities, such as picking and moving objects and flying through space. Collaborative, interactive controls such as cutting planes, windowing, and a color lookup table are accessible to all the users over the network. Object-orientated structure makes it easy to add new functions into the application.

Changes in windowing and cutting planes are distributed through a transmission control protocol channel to other participants who are involved in the tele-immersive environment. Streaming audio is supported in the environment through a user datagram protocol port. Participants who are at different ends of the world can see each other, work on the same data set, and talk to each other in real time.

The tele-immersive system includes stereo vision, viewer-centered perspective, a sense of touch, and collaboration. Both volume rendering and haptic rendering are processing-intensive. To achieve optimized performance, this system includes a dual-processor PC, NVIDIA's high-performance graphics card, fast volume rendering with 3D texture mapping, and a multi-threading architecture.

A rendering thread updates the stereo display of the volumetric data at about 20 fps. A haptic rendering thread calculates the force feedback at a rate of 1 kHz, and a much slower user interface thread handles user commands. Patient CT data and transformation matrices need to be shared among threads. A mutual exclusion algorithm (mutex) locking mechanism has been carefully designed to avoid data access conflicts. The result is an augmented reality system that has no noticeable latency between visual feedback and haptic feedback.

The CAVE library (CAVELib®) [3] is an application programming interface that provides a software environment/toolkit for developing VR applications. CAVELib is used in the tele-immersive radiological application, and it is used to interface with the tracking and the rendering system. A C++ class has been created to handle the display window and the user interaction. The class is able to process multiple volumes.

The software system is designed with portability in mind, and the development tools used in this project can run on both Linux and Windows platforms. The software has been successfully built on Fedora and SUSE Linux machines. The software system has also been successfully built and installed on a portable

Shuttle® PC running Fedora Linux. This is useful when we need to set up a portable system for field consultation and demonstration.

The software system has been configured to be able to run in different working environments. It can be used on a PARIS with CAVELib and haptics support. It can also run on a PC with a normal monitor. It can be built with or without network support. It can also be built with or without haptics support, which may be necessary when it is used on a physician's desktop VR system when a haptics device is not available.

5.7
Conclusions

Instead of limiting medical volume visualization to one geographic location, the combination of teleconferencing, telepresence, and VR allows this radiological tele-immersive environment to enable geographically distributed clinicians to intuitively interact with the same medical volumetric models, point, gesture, converse, and see each other. This environment brings together clinicians at different geographic locations to participate in tele-immersive consultation and collaboration.

This comprehensive tele-immersive system includes a variety of VR devices, such as a conference-room-sized system for tele-immersive small-group consultation and an inexpensive, easily deployable networked desktop VR system for surgical consultation, evaluation, and collaboration.

This system has been used to design patient-specific cranial implants with precise fit. It can also be used in consultation, preoperative planning, surgical simulation, postoperative evaluation, education, and large-scale health emergencies.

Summary

- It is important to make patient-specific data quickly available and usable to many specialists at different geographical sites.
- A tele-immersive radiological system has been developed for remote consultation, surgical preplanning, postoperative evaluation, and education.
- Tele-immersive devices

  - PARIS
  - C-Wall
  - Physician's personal VR display
  - ImmersaDesk

- Volume rendering
- Cluster-based visualization of large-scale volumetric data
- Tele-immersive collaboration
- System implementation

Acknowledgments

This publication was made possible, in part, by grant no. N01-LM-3-3507 from the National Library of Medicine, National Institutes of Health.

References

1. Ai Z et al (2002) Tele-immersive medical educational environment. Stud Health Technol Inform 85:24–30
2. Cabral B, Cam N, Foran J (1994) Accelerated volume rendering and tomographic reconstruction using texture mapping hardware. In: Proceedings of the 1994 symposium on Volume visualization. Tysons Corner 91–98
3. Cruz-Neira C, Sandin DJ, DeFanti TA (1993) Surround-screen projection-based virtual reality: the design and implementation of the CAVE. In: Proceedings of SIGGRAPH 93. ACM New York, NY, USA, pp 135–142
4. Czernuszenko M et al (1997) The ImmersaDesk and infinity wall projection-based virtual reality displays. Comput Graph 31:46–49
5. Hendin O, John NW, Shocet O (1998) Medical volume rendering over the WWW using VRML and Java. In: Proceedings of medicine meets virtual reality. Edited by James D. Westwood, Helene M. Hoffman, Don Stredney and Suzanne J. Weghorst. Published by IOS/Ohmsha Press - Amsterdam/Berlin/Oxford/Tokyo/Washington, DC, p 409
6. http://www.sensable.com/haptic-phantom-desktop.htm. Last Accessed 02 May 2008
7. Kajiya JT, Herzen BPV (1984) Ray tracing volume densities. In: Proceedings of the SIGGRAPH'84. 18:165–174
8. Leigh J, Johnson AE, DeFanti TA (1997) Global tele-immersion: better than being there. In: Proceedings of ICAT'97 Tokyo, Japan, Dec 3-5
9. Leigh J, Johnson A, DeFanti T, Bailey S, and Grossman R (1999) A tele-immersive environment for collaborative exploratory analysis of massive data sets. In: Proceedings of ASCI 99, Heijen, the Netherlands
10. Leigh J, Yee O, Schonfeld D, Ansari R, et al (2001) Adaptive networking for tele-immersion. In: Proceedings of the Immersive Projection Technology/Eurographics Virtual Environments Workshop (IPT/EGVE), May 16–18, Stuttgart, Germany
11. Magallon M, Hopf M, Ertl T (2001) Parallel volume rendering using PC graphics hardware. In: Ninth pacific conference on computer graphics and applications (Pacific Graphics'01)
12. Pearl RK, Evenhouse R, Rasmussen M, et al (1999) The virtual pelvic floor, a tele-immersive educational environment. Proc AMIA Symp 345–348
13. Porter T, Duff T (1984) Compositing digital images. Comput Graph 18: 253–259
14. Rasmussen M et al (1998) The virtual temporal bone, a tele-immersive educational environment. Future Gener Comput Syst 125–130

15. Rezk-Salama C, et al (2000) Interactive Volume Rendering on Standard PC Graphics Hardware Using Multi-Textures and Multi-Stage Rasterization, 2000 Siggraph/Eurographics Workshop Graphics Hardware, ACM Press, New York, pp 109–118
16. Schroeder W, Martin K, Lorensen B (1996) The visualization toolkit: an object-oriented approach to 3D graphics. Prentice-Hall, Englewood Cliffs
17. Silverstein J, Rubenstein J, Millman A, and Panko W (1998) Web-based segmentation and display of 3-dimensional radiologic image data. In: Westwood JD, Hoffman HM, Stredney D, and Weghorst SJ, eds, Proceedings of Medicine Meets Virtual Reality, San Diego, Amsterdam, Jan, IOS Press, 6:53–59
18. Stredney D, Crawfis R, Wiet GJ, Sessanna D, Shareef N, and Bryan J (1999) Interactive volume visualizations for synchronous and asynchronous remote collaboration. In: Westwood J.D. et al. (ed.) Medicine Meets Virtual Reality, IOS Press, 344–350

6

Use of a Radiology Picture Archiving and Communication System to Catalogue Photographic Images

James E. Silberzweig and Azita S. Khorsandi

Abstract Visible-light images can be easily and successfully archived using a system primarily intended for radiographic images. Extending the coverage of a single interconnected picture archiving and communication system to all image-producing services can potentially improve overall hospital-wide workflow.

6.1
Introduction

Advances in medicine and complexity of patients' illnesses have both required a multidisciplinary approach to treatment. This requires accessible and up-to-date medical records to be shared by all the physicians caring for the patient. This has led to the development oft the electronic medical record system.

Most modern radiology departments utilize a picture archiving and communication system (PACS) for radiographic image and report viewing and historical archival. The PACS also features workflow management including organizing studies, presenting them in a consistent manner in the form of work lists and keeping track of study status. A PACS typically consists of an archive device, diagnostic viewing stations for radiologists, clinical review by physicians, and servers to distribute the images throughout the hospital network.

There are many specialties beyond radiology that produce medically relevant nonradiographic images that require archiving and may benefit from imaging workflow management. Specialties including cardiology; dermatology; ophthalmology; surgery; ear, nose, and throat; pathology; gastroenterology; and surgery can all benefit from implementation of a PACS. Imaging modalities include endoscopy with video, microscopy, and photographic (visible-light) images. Some of these specialties use a local database system with limited capabilities. Images frequently cannot be exported or retrieved from external sources. Most current electronic medical record systems do not have the capability of storage of images for all medical specialties in a single location. A radiology PACS can potentially function as a model for a multispecialty PACS storing all diagnostic images acquired within a hospital [1].

The use of radiology department PACS tools can be extended beyond conventional radiology imaging to include secondary document acquisition, such as scanned documents, including prescriptions and patient questionnaires. Our radiology practice was able to use a conventional PACS primarily intended for radiographic images for viewing and archiving of photographic visible-light images. Our experience with archiving visible-light images is an example of how nonradiology images can be incorporated into a radiology PACS. Extending the coverage of a single interconnected PACS to other image-producing services can potentially improve overall hospital-wide workflow.

6.2
Experience with Documenting Venous Insufficiency

Recent developments in the percutaneous treatment of venous insufficiency have allowed evaluation and management of lower-extremity varicose veins/ venous insufficiency to become a significant component of many interventional radiology practices [5, 6]. Typically, the documentation of an initial clinical evaluation of a patient with lower-extremity venous insufficiency includes a consultation report, a lower-extremity venous duplex sonogram, and photographs of the lower extremities. Data may be stored in a hard-copy file folder or a computer database. Among the limitations enforced by maintaining a hard-copy system are the inadequate capabilities of image backup and redundancy, high image-developing expenses, and the inability to access patient data from any remote site, if needed.

Over a 20-month period, our practice evaluated 104 patients with lower-extremity venous insufficiency, lower-extremity varicose veins, and/or telangiectasias [8]. Clinical evaluations were performed in a freestanding outpatient interventional radiology facility. Clinical evaluation documentation consisted of a consultation report, a venous duplex sonogram, and photographs of the lower extremities.

Photographs were taken using a commercially available digital camera. A neutral-colored background was used. Automatic flash was employed with standard overhead fluorescent room lighting. Photographs were taken at an average of 2 m from the patient. Photographs of the patient's lower extremities included four views: anterior, posterior, lateral right, and lateral left. The consultation report and duplex ultrasound reports with images were archived in the radiology department PACS. The images and reports were archived using a method similar to the method used to process any other type of radiology study (ultrasound; computed tomography, CT; magnetic resonance imaging, MRI; nuclear medicine; mammography; etc.).

Following that, the photographic images were transferred from the camera to a conventional desktop personal computer using a standard such as Joint Photographic Experts Group (JPEG) file format using a USB card reader. The images were then manipulated (rotated and cropped) as needed using Microsoft Office Picture Manager (Microsoft, Redmond, WA, USA). The images were then transferred back from the desktop computer to a USB 2.0 flash drive and uploaded to the PACS using the tools of a dedicated PACS workstation (Horizon Review Station, version 4.6.1, McKesson Medical Imaging, Vancouver, BC, Canada). The PACS encapsulated the JPEG images with a wrapper. The wrapper created digital imaging and communications in medicine (DICOM) objects from the non-DICOM JPEG files. The photographic image files were archived with each patient's clinical consultation report and sonogram.

The PACS display included the photographic images along with the demographic information including the patient's name, date, medical record number, examination type, gender, and patient's age (Fig. 6.1). Images could

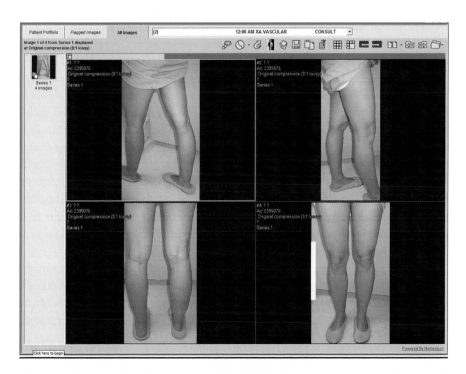

Fig. 6.1. The screenshot demonstrates a photographic image on a picture archiving and communication system of a 33-year-old woman with lower-extremity venous insufficiency/varicose veins. The screen includes the photographic images as well as demographic information and date

also be subsequently exported to a compact disc (CD) or a USB 2.0 flash drive for transfer to a computer linked to a paper color printer for generation of hard copy.

The location and extent of venous disease is documented by written description in the consultation report, by a duplex sonogram, and with photographs. Findings including varicosities, telangiectasias, skin color changes, and ulcerations are readily demonstrated in photographs. Photographic documentation can be used as a guide to evaluate treatment progress for both the treating physician and the patient. Additionally, insurance carriers may request photographic documentation.

In our practice, prior to the implementation of photographic image transfer to the PACS, all photographic images were transferred from the camera to a conventional desktop computer as a JPEG file. The files were either stored on the computer hard drive with intermittent backup made onto CD or printed on paper and filed in the patient's hard-copy folder. These photographs were archived separately from the radiology department PACS data.

Limitations of our previous photographic image archive system included the inability to access the photographs from a remote workstation, limited backup capability, and the requirement to access separate databases to evaluate a single patient's clinical data. Additionally, a separately named computer file folder needed to be created for each patient.

In our experience, the use of our PACS for photographic image storage has been quite reliable. The PACS has been widely used in our radiology department daily practice routine for the past 5 years. On a typical weekday, over 1,200 radiology examinations are sent to the radiology department PACS. Modalities capable of sending images to the PACS include CT, MRI, interventional radiology, sonography, nuclear medicine, computed radiography, and digital mammography. Image storage capacity with this system is virtually limitless. Data are stored on a series of network servers' hard drives, with a backup archive in an offsite location. Additional data backup on tape is performed as the disaster recovery solution, giving the site a three-tier redundancy of image archive.

The use of a PACS at other medical centers has been extended to manage all medical images acquired within the hospital, including nonradiology imaging applications such as endoscopy and microscopy images in addition to photographic images obtained in dermatology and ophthalmology departments [1, 3].

Most PACS can import files from multiple formats, including JPEG, Tagged Image File Format (TIFF), and DICOM. One report demonstrated experience with the ability of a PACS to integrate outside imaging studies on a recordable CD and transfer the data into a local PACS [9].

We used the JPEG format for image acquisition and transfer to the PACS. In general, the major advantage for using TIFF over JPEG files is that TIFF gives the best-quality image because it is uncompressed (lossless). However, use of TIFF comes at the expense of large image size [4]. Digital camera images of patients acquired in JPEG format have been shown to be reliable for plastic surgery and vascular surgery [2, 7].

6.3
Conclusion

We believe that photographic image transfer to a PACS can be used by nearly any varicose vein/venous insufficiency treatment practice that has access to a conventional radiology PACS. The system provides access to a reliable, secure, virtually limitless image and clinical data archive, offering the clinician a complete, chronological view of the patient clinical record. Our experience serves as one example of how nonradiology images can potentially be incorporated into a radiology PACS. Integration of the varied needs of multiple clinical services requires a system that is robust and can provide specialized attention and flexibility to diverse workflow requirements.

A unified collaborative approach to the electronic record for medical imaging would allow a more cohesive, comprehensive, and precise evaluation of a patient rather than treating the patient in multiple pieces.

Summary

- Visible-light images can be easily and successfully archived using a system primarily intended for radiographic images.
- Extending the coverage of a single interconnected PACS to all image-producing services can potentially improve overall hospital-wide workflow.

References

1. Bandon D, Lovis C, Geissbuhler A, Vallee JP (2005) Enterprise-wide PACS: beyond radiology, an architecture to manage all medical images. Acad Radiol 12:1000–1009
2. Galdino GM, Vogel JE, Vander Kolk CA (2001) Standardizing digital photography: it's not all in the eye of the beholder. Plast Reconstr Surg 108:1334–1344
3. Kuzmak PM, Dayhoff RE (2000) The use of digital imaging and communications in medicine (DICOM) in the integration of imaging into the electronic patient record at the Department of Veterans Affairs. J Digit Imaging 13:133–137

4. LaBerge JM, Andriole KP (2003) Digital image processing: a primer for JVIR authors and readers: part 1: the fundamentals. J Vasc Interv Radiol 14:1223–1230

5. Merchant RF, Pichot O, Closure Study Group (2005) Long-term outcomes of endovenous radiofrequency obliteration of saphenous reflux as a treatment for superficial venous insufficiency. J Vasc Surg 42:502–509

6. Min RJ, Khilnani N, Zimmet SE (2003) Endovenous laser treatment of saphenous vein reflux: long-term results. J Vasc Interv Radiol 14:991–996

7. Murphy RX Jr, Bain MA, Wasser TE, Wilson E, Okunski WJ (2006) The reliability of digital imaging in the remote assessment of wounds: defining a standard. Ann Plast Surg 56:431–436

8. Silberzweig JE, Khorsandi AS, El-Shayal T, Abiri MM (2007) The use of a picture archiving and communication system to catalogue visible-light photographic images. J Vasc Interv Radiol 18:577–579

9. van Ooijen PM, Guignot J, Mevel G, Oudkerk M (2005) Incorporating out-patient data from CD-R into the local PACS using DICOM worklist features. J Digit Imaging 18:196–202

7

Teleradiology with DICOM E-mail

Peter Mildenberger

Abstract Transmission of radiological studies requires high quality for reporting and therefore for the transfer of digital imaging and communication in medicine (DICOM) objects. DICOM e-mail, as defined by the DICOM Committee, has this potential. Additional attention has to be given to security aspects, especially encryption. There is a national approach regarding all these aspects in Germany, now providing open-source-based and commercial products.

7.1
Introduction

Teleradiology has been known for many years. In the beginning, all companies had their own proprietary solutions. There was no interoperability between different products. This was no problem for a bilateral communication between a center and one or more partners. But this was a barrier for communication between different independent users [1].

Therefore, this issue was picked up by digital imaging and communication in medicine (DICOM), and a discussion on possible solutions started within the DICOM Committee in 2000. The DICOM Committee is working on interoperability issues in different medical imaging areas, and DICOM is the world standard for medical imaging [2]. The analysis for different technical solutions showed that an e-mail-based solution would fit best in IT environments. The final paper (DICOM Supplement 54) was published in 2003 defining the DICOM multipurpose Internet mail extension (MIME) type.

This approach was grabbed by a group in Germany in the same year, forming an alliance between users and vendors supported by the German Roentgen Society. The aim of this group was to establish a concept for a secure use of DICOM e-mail with Internet connections. This was necessary because DICOM Supplement 54 does not include security aspects such as encryption or signature.

7.2
Technical Aspects

The DICOM MIME Type describes how to include attached files as "parts" into Internet e-mail. These may be sent by protocols such as simple mail transfer protocol (SMTP). This solution is intended to improve or enable the use of DICOM network protocols for different applications, such as:

- Hospital-to-doctor DICOM object (image) distribution
- Exchange of DICOM objects for testing purposes
- DICOM object distribution for education, scientific cooperation, and contract research
- Interpretation by professionals at home

The aspects of such applications are better integration with desktop applications, moderate expectations of reliability and conformance, less centralized control over the system's setup, and configuration.

The DICOM MIME Type concept covers two levels:

1. The Application/dicom MIME Type for the DICOM file level
2. The Multipart/mixed MIME Type for the file-set level

This application uses the normal media storage service class. A compatible solution has to support either the *File Set Creator* role and/or the *File Set Reader* role. In such a file set, a DICOMDIR (table of contents) may be included.

As part of the DICOM supplement there are already some recommendations regarding security or interoperability considerations.

This DICOM-based approach for a communication had been picked up by the German group in the year of the publication (2003). This group of about 15 different users and vendors analyzed different technical solutions for a secure and interoperable communication between independent organizations (hospitals and physicians' practices), including secure shell, virtual private networks (VPNs), secure file transfer protocol, and others.

The consensus in this group was to find a general platform for sending and receiving images with related information based on international standards and compliant with national and international law. The solution should be easy to integrate in normal picture archiving and communication system (PACS) environment. Interoperabilty tests analog to the Integrating Healthcare Enterprise (IHE) connectathons were held.

Very soon there was a consensus to use DICOM MIME Type and to add some regulations for encryption, signature, firewall restrictions, and support of multipart messages. A central discussion was held regarding the encryption of the e-mails. Of course there are recommendations for use of secure MIME (S/MIME), but, in fact, in Germany there is no established infrastructure with X509 certificates (public key infrastructure), which are required hereafter, and there were some problems with the interoperability of open-source-based S/MIME tools. This led to use of a pretty good privacy based approach with OpenPGP. This is very well known and accepted by official authorities too (Federal Office for Information Security in Germany). Of course there are other countries that have already introduced a common security infrastructure for health-care professionals (e.g., France and Austria); in these countries the use of S/MIME is established. The integration of non-DICOM data is possible in principle too. This is necessary to add patient information.

More details on the technical aspects can be found at http://www.tele-x-standard.de or in [4]. The secure DICOM e-mail concept has been accepted and recommended by the German Roentgen Society.

7.3
Experiences

Different protocols are used for secure teleradiology connections. For example, with a VPN problems could arise with networks of many partners or partners who are members of different VPNs. Similar restrictions could be found with HTTPS-based image distribution. Workflow integration is less comfortable, and the waiting time will be higher than with the DICOM e-mail approach.

As of today there are about seven different vendors supporting this concept in Germany. In these solutions, users will find a seamless integration in their workplaces. They have to decide which study, series, or images should be send and to whom (Fig. 7.1). The following process of sending the DICOM objects to the teleradiology gateway, encryption, and signature is completely automated and does not require handling by the radiologist or technician. On the other hand, for the destination, it is vice versa. Images will be decrypted and sent to predefined PACS servers or workstations. All this could be coupled with notification per fax, e-mail, or SMS.

These solutions from different vendors are compatible. Many installations with different products on both sites are in use already. Interoperability using this DICOM e-mail approach can be assured owing to the regulations and testing done by this group in Germany. In one region of Germany (Baden-Württemberg), DICOM-e-mail has become the standard teleradiology protocol as a result of legal advice from the official authorities [3], now serving more than 50 hospitals and other partners.

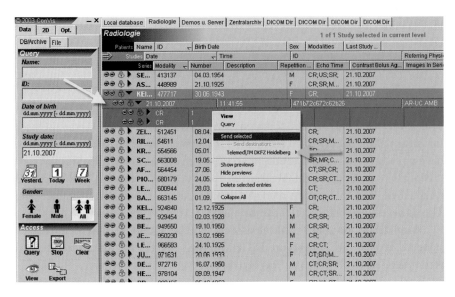

Fig. 7.1. Example of a standard picture archiving and communication system workplace with selected images (*yellow arrow*) and teleradiology destination (*green arrow*)

The use of an Internet connection could cause problems owing to instability, bandwidth, spam e-mail, viruses, or other reasons. Therefore, users should try to prevent these possible problems using firewalls and backup solutions. Viruses and spam e-mails have not been found to be a real problem in the German sites, because direct SMTP connections with dedicated e-mail servers are in use and the clients do not execute any attachment. International partners are already included with this DICOM e-mail approach.

In the future, different developments could be expected. There is an increasing interest in DICOM e-mail in the USA, especially by the American Dental Association. Current developments of GnuPGP tools include the implementation of S/MIME. This could help to harmonize the different approaches in various countries regarding encryption. And overall there is, first, discussion within the IHE on workflow concepts of teleradiology; this will help in international standardization in this topic.

7.4
Conclusion

DICOM e-mail is an excellent basis for building interoperable teleradiology solutions. Special attention must be given to security aspects, especially encryption. A regulation for these topics has been provided in Germany by a group under the umbrella of the German Roentgen Society. Different open-source-based and commercial solutions are available and used routinely.

Summary

- Transmission of radiological studies requires high quality for reporting and therefore for the transfer of DICOM objects.
- DICOM e-mail, as defined by the DICOM Committee, has this potential.
- Additional attention has to be given to security aspects, especially encryption.

There is a national approach regarding all these aspects in Germany, now providing open-source-based and commercial products.

References

1. http://en.wikipedia.org/wiki/. Last date Accessed 01 May 2008
2. http://medical.nema.org/
3. http://www.teleradiologie-rnd.de/
4. Weisser G, Walz M, Ruggiero S et al (2006) Standardization of teleradiology using DICOM e-mail: recommendations of the German Radiology Society. Eur Radiol 16(3):753–758

8

Teleradiology Multimedia Messaging Service in the Provision of Emergency Neurosurgical Service

Wai Hoe Ng, Ernest Wang, and Ivan Ng

Abstract Neurosurgery is limited by the availability of highly trained professionals and resources. Interpretation of scan images is highly vital for accurate diagnosis and institution of appropriate treatment, which can have significant impact on patient care and outcome. Currently, there are various methods of transmitting important scan images to experienced medical staff for accurate interpretation. Multimedia messaging service (MMS) technology is a readily available, simple, and cost-effective method for the transmission of scan images. The use of MMS technology in emergency neurosurgery services has been effective in enhancing the confidence of neurosurgeons in clinical decision making, reducing the need for hospital call-back, and improving patient care.

8.1
Background

Optimal provision of medical service is contingent on the accurate assessment of patients, sound interpretation of relevant laboratory and imaging investigations, and the institution of prompt and appropriate therapy.

In the emergent setting, the processes are similar but may at times need to be prioritized on the basis of the level of urgency and the ability to perform specialized tests in a timely fashion.

Neurosurgery is a highly specialized specialty, which is limited by the availability of sufficiently trained and accredited specialists and also the provision of highly cost-intensive equipment. In addition, a neurosurgical service does not exist in isolation but is supported by similarly highly trained specialists such as neurologists, neuroradiologists, neuroanesthetists, and neurointensive care specialists.

As such, neurosurgical units are usually based in large major metropolitan tertiary hospitals and provide neurosurgical cover to large segments of the metropolitan population as well as district and country hospitals, which may be located at considerable distance.

Unfortunately, neurosurgical emergencies form a significant proportion of a tertiary neurosurgical service. These potentially life threatening conditions encountered mandate prompt and accurate diagnosis and the rapid institution of definitive therapy to reduce neurological mortality and morbidity.

Two major issues arise from this issue of emergent treatment:

1. *Need for accurate scan interpretation*: The scan image (computed tomography, CT, or magnetic resonance imaging, MRI) is arguably the single most critical investigation in the emergent setting for neurosurgery. Rapid institution of appropriate treatment is entirely dependent on the accurate interpretation of scan images and assessment of the clinical status of the patient.

   Most neurosurgical units are operated on a two-tier system after standard working hours. The in-house service is normally run by a middle-level staff. The middle-level staff is conventionally a neurosurgeon-in-training (registrar or resident), and the senior staff (consultant or attending) is normally consulted on issues through telephonic conversations.

   The intricacy of neuroanatomy and unfamiliarity with interpretation of CT or MRI images by the in-house staff may potentially result in erroneous or missed diagnosis. This can obviously lead to devastating adverse effects as appropriate therapy may be delayed. A system of quality control in scan interpretation can, therefore, minimize or eliminate this problem.

2. *Evaluation of need for emergent transfer to a neurosurgical unit from a district or country hospital*: Neurosurgical emergencies regrettably frequently occur in areas without access to a neurosurgical unit. These patients are normally evacuated to a district or country hospital where the initial assessment and resuscitation are performed. If a neurosurgical problem is identified, the attending clinicians then need to decide on the urgency of transfer.

   Traditionally, patients are assessed at the district or country hospital, and the need and urgency for transfer are made via information conveyed by a tele-phonic consultation with the attending neurosurgeon. This system is fraught with problems, as vital information critical to optimal patient care may not be conveyed accurately or promptly [18].

   Scan images coupled with relevant clinical information arguably provide the single most important information to facilitate prompt and appropriate patient management. Accurate clinical assessment can normally be performed at the district hospitals. Most district hospitals now also have access to a CT scan. However, familiarity with scan interpretation may be encountered, necessitating a system of scan transfer for accurate assessment.

It is especially crucial that the scans are interpreted accurately so that prompt and appropriate treatment can be commenced. The urgency for transfer is also largely based on the scan findings and clinical condition of the patient. It is essential to assess the need for transfer appropriately, as premature transfer before adequate resuscitation can lead to adverse outcomes [6]. Delay in transfer due to unrecognized potentially serious disease conditions can also similarly result in poor outcome. There are also instances of unnecessary transfer to the tertiary neurosurgical unit, which results in inappropriate and inefficient utilization of scarce resources [3].

A system of image transfer of appropriate and relevant scans from less experienced medical staff to senior staff can overcome all the current inadequacies in the provision of emergency neurosurgical services and in turn translate into superior patient care and outcome.

8.2
Global Experience

There are many inherent problems associated with the traditional telephonic consultation. In the early 1980s, Gentleman and Jennett examined 150 comatose patients with head injury transferred to their center from neighboring hospitals and found that 18 patients had respiratory arrest on arrival and two patients actually died on arrival. This highlights the fact that interhospital transfer is potentially hazardous, especially if clinical assessment is inadequate [18].

The shortcomings of interhospital patient transfer have resulted in the impetus for the application of modern teleradiology technology for the management of neurosurgical emergencies, which was pioneered in the early 1990s in Europe and the USA.

The implementation of one such early image transfer systems used to link scanners within the Oxford region in the UK was reported in 1990 [13]. CT scan images for patients not requiring immediate transfer, based on clinical examination, are transferred from the regional hospital to the tertiary neurosurgical unit in Oxford via the dedicated Image Link, which was a machine that transferred scan images via telephone. The use of this Image Link system resulted in substantial improvements in management of emergency neurosurgery referrals, cost-effectiveness of neurosurgical and ambulance services, and more speedy interhospital transfer.

Since then, the use of such a telephone/modem-based image transfer system has been implemented in many neurosurgical units around the world, including in Hong Kong [8, 16, 19], Poland [7], Spain [15], Norway [17], and South Africa [11]. Analysis of the experience by the various units has shown unequivocal results that the technique has enhanced patient care, accelerated patient transfer, reduced unnecessary transfer, and led to more rational use of valuable and scarce resources. In the Norwegian experience, image transfer was considered beneficial in 93% of cases. Avoidance of unnecessary patient transfer, changes of treatment at the referring hospital on the advice of the neurosurgeon, and initiation of emergency transfer occurred in 34, 42, and 13% of cases, respectively.

In Hong Kong, teleradiology initiatives have varied between powerful workstations using dedicated data lines as part of an academic information technology project and commercially available systems using standard personal computers (PCs) and telephone lines. The neurosurgical unit at the Chinese University utilizes a PC-based teleradiology system, which enables CT scan images to be transmitted via telephone lines directly to a PC in the neurosurgical unit or to a portable notebook computer attended to by the on-call neurosurgeon [16].

An alternative to the telephone/modem-based system is the use of a charge coupled device (CCD) scanner to digitize CT or MRI scan images and transmit the digitized images via integrated systems digital network (ISDN) lines [9]. Each CCD is a silicon-based, light-sensitive device that generates electrons in proportion to the amount of incident light over a defined period of time. A picture is then formed when the number of electrons within each pixel in the CCD is converted into a digital value. The images are then sent to the regional neurosurgical unit via leased data lines and B-channel ISDN lines, at 128 kilobits/s. The system runs on PCs with the Microsoft Windows operating system. This system has been utilized on a national level in Ireland, with a population of 3.5 million, and is served by only two neurosurgical centers, located in Cork and Dublin. The widespread installation of CT scanners in the regional hospitals coupled with the ease of use of the system has resulted in a cost-effective system with superior image quality and widespread physician acceptance.

Digital image creation with a hand-held digital camera is followed by electronic mail (e-mail) transfer across the Internet by using a local Internet service provider. The original CT scan images are interpreted by a radiologist, and the interpretation of the distant CT scan images (e-mail-attached images) is done by the neurosurgeon and comparison is subsequently made with the radiologist's formal interpretation. Apple and Schmidt [1] evaluated 30 abnormal CT scans and found that there was a difference in diagnosis on only one image and that there was no visibly demonstrable difference in image quality between digital and hard-copy images. The image transfer time to the neurosurgeon's computer for viewing averaged only 15 min. This hand-held, inexpensive digital camera and e-mail system can therefore be a valuable alternative to more sophisticated teleradiology techniques.

Recent advances in modern information and communication technology have provided rapid and high-resolution audiovisual imaging at acceptable costs, thereby providing the additional option of video consultation. Teleradiology can therefore be augmented with videoconferencing facilities to provide an additional avenue for patient evaluation.

The comparative impact of video consultation on emergency neurosurgical referrals was investigated by Wong et al. [19]. A randomized controlled trial was conducted, whereby consecutive patients from the district general hospital requiring emergency neurosurgical consultation were recruited and stratified into three diagnosis groups: (1) head injury group, (2) hemorrhagic stroke group, and (3) miscellaneous group.

Within each disease category, patients were further randomized by double-sealed envelopes into three modes of consultation:

1. *Telephonic consultation*: The referring physician was required to telephone and discuss in detail with the on-call neurosurgeon the case history, physical signs, and relevant investigation.
2. *Teleradiology*: Images were transferred from the district general hospital to the neurosurgical center via Windows-based software (Multiview Teleradiology for Windows, version 2.0; MERGE EMED, Milwaukee, WI, USA) in addition to the telephonic consultation.
3. *Video consultation*: Patients and any relevant radiology images could be viewed at the same time, using low-cost commercial real-time interactive videoconferencing equipment (Polycom View Station; Polycom, San Jose, CA, USA) installed in the accident and emergency departments of the hospitals, connected by an ISDN line transmitting information at 256 kilobits/s.

Over a 3-year period, 710 patients were recruited. Teleradiology and video consultation showed a definite advantage in diagnostic accuracy over traditional telephonic consultation (89.1 and 87.7% compared with 63.8%; $p < 0.001$). However, the duration of consultation was longer for teleradiology and video consultation than for telephonic consultation (1.01 and 1.3 h compared with 0.70 h). There was a trend toward more favorable outcome (61%; $p = 0.1$) and reduced mortality (25%; $p = 0.025$) in teleradiology compared with telephonic consultation (54 and 34%, respectively) and video consultation (54 and 33%, respectively). Video consultation, however, had a high failure rate of 30%. Teleradiology and video consultation can therefore provide higher levels of diagnostic accuracy and improve patient outcome compared with traditional telephonic consultation. However, video consultation offers no additional advantage over teleradiology.

8.3
Multimedia Messaging Service

Multimedia messaging service (MMS) is the evolution of short message service (which is a text-only messaging technology for mobile networks) and allows for the transmission and receipt of graphics, video, and audio clips.

MMS mobile phone technology is prevalent and readily available. It offers a simple, cheap, quick, and effective solution to the problem of scan interpretation. An MMS takes only a few minutes to send and receive and allows senior physicians to view important images and make important clinical decisions to enhance patient management in an emergency situation. The technology is already in widespread use and can be seamlessly and rapidly be implemented in the clinical arena.

The first report of the application and usefulness of the MMS image transfer system was recorded in 2002 in neurosurgery patients [20]. The main advantages of the system lie in the low cost and ease of handling for transmission of images to remote areas and between hospitals. In spite of the small dimensions of the monitor, the images were of sufficiently high quality. Since the first report, MMS has also been used in the evaluation of emergency ear, nose, and throat radiological investigations [5] and to facilitate the referral of musculoskeletal limb injuries to a tertiary referral center [2].

Similarly, in our neurosurgical unit at the National Neuroscience Institute, Singapore, MMS technology has been utilized in the routine management of neurosurgical patients since 2006 to enhance patient care [14].

A designated mobile phone (with video graphics array, VGA, camera and MMS capabilities) was provided to the neurosurgery registrar on call. This designated mobile phone is always held by the registrar on call. All consultants had personal mobile phones that are MMS-enabled.

Relevant representative CT/MRI images are taken directly with the VGA camera on the mobile phone from the picture archiving and communication system off the computer screen (Figs. 8.1, 8.2). When only scan films are available, the images can be taken off the light box. On average, three to four images per CT/MRI series are captured and transmitted to the consultant neurosurgeon for expert opinion. The total time for the registrar to acquire these three to four images is about 60 s. Each image is then sent as a "picture message," with another 60 s before the consultant receives the picture message. In total, it takes 3–5 min for the consultant to view all the relevant scans.

A questionnaire (Table 8.1) to ascertain the following information was given to all senior- and middle-level staff (total number 12) after a 12-month trial period to validate the effectiveness of the MMS technology:

- How frequently was the MMS system utilized?
- Did the MMS system facilitate the neurosurgical staff in clinical decision making?
- Was the quality of the MMS images sufficient to make sound clinical decisions?
- Did the use of MMS reduce the need for hospital call-back for the consultant neurosurgeon on call?

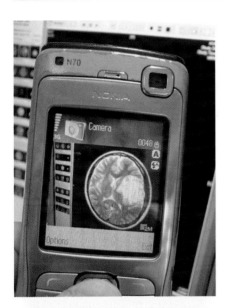

Fig. 8.1. Taking a multimedia messaging service (MMS) image off the computer screen

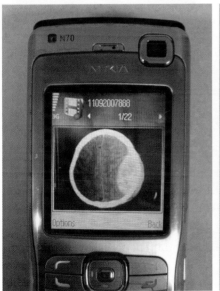

a

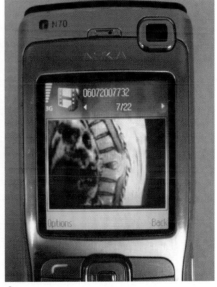

b

Fig. 8.2. a MMS image showing a large extradural hematoma from head injury. **b** MMS image showing a vertebral tumor causing significant spinal cord compression

The findings of the questionnaire demonstrated that MMS was utilized in approximately 50% of on-call roster. It was generally found to be more useful by the senior staff compared with the junior staff and significantly increased their level of confidence in clinical decision making and reduced their need to

Table 8.1. Questionnaire on multimedia messaging service *(MMS)*

Consultant

1. How frequently do you use MMS when you are on call?
   - <25%
   - 25–50%
   - 51–75%
   - >75%

2. Did the use of MMS improve your level of confidence in clinical decision making?
   - No difference
   - Slight difference
   - Moderate difference
   - Significant difference

3. Did the use of MMS reduce the need for on-call call-back?
   - Yes
   - No

4. Would viewing the actual scans versus the MMS images change your initial clinical decision?
   - Yes
   - No

Registrar

1. How frequently do you use MMS when you are on call?
   - <25%
   - 25–50%
   - 51–75%
   - >75%

2. Did the use of MMS improve your level of confidence in clinical decision making?
   - No difference
   - Slight difference
   - Moderate difference
   - Significant difference

3. Did the use of MMS provide important input from attending consultant?
   - No difference
   - Slight difference
   - Moderate difference
   - Significant difference

return to hospital to evaluate patients or scans. Significantly, nearly all senior staff felt that the MMS images were of sufficient quality for them to make an accurate assessment, and viewing the actual scans the next day made no difference in their clinical decision.

8.4
Conclusion

Emergency neurosurgery services must necessarily be provided on a 24-h basis. Outside standard working hours, the provision of emergency services is conventionally provided in a two-tiered fashion, with the in-house staff manned by middle-level physicians (usually neurosurgeons-in-training) who would consult the senior physicians on more complex clinical problems via telephonic consultations. Physicians in a district hospital also need to arrange transfer of patients to the relevant tertiary center with neurosurgical facilities via telephonic consultations. The inherent shortcomings of telephonic consultation may have significant impact on patient care.

Accurate scan interpretation is vital for the diagnosis of neurosurgical emergencies, as prompt diagnosis and rapid institution of definitive treatment can potentially be life-saving. The complexity of neuroanatomy and unfamiliarity with interpretation of CT or MRI images by the in-house staff and a nonneurosurgical specialist in a district hospital can result in erroneous or missed diagnosis with adverse effects, as appropriate therapy may be delayed.

The use of teleradiology can overcome this problem, as the on-call team can send relevant images to the senior physician, who can then review the images. Integration with PCs and networking with teleradiology systems are now possible, although the installation of such systems in every consultant's household becomes impractical and expensive. Image transfer systems based on e-mail, ISDN, and other techniques have also been proposed [8, 10, 12, 16] and are certainly useful and have been used to assess the need of interhospital transfer of neurosurgical patients [9, 11, 13, 16]. The disadvantages of such systems lie in the need for costly equipment, more intensive training, and a static workstation to view incoming images.

The MMS mobile phone system offers a simple, cheap, quick, and effective solution to the problem of scan interpretation. An MMS takes only a few minutes to send and receive and allows senior physicians to view important images and make important clinical decisions to enhance patient management in an emergency situation. The technology is already in widespread use and can be seamlessly and rapidly implemented in the clinical arena. Significantly, it enables the senior staff to access the images from anywhere without the need for a workstation.

This technology therefore has great promise in the area of interhospital transfer of neurosurgical patients and in the optimization of the delivery of care within tertiary referral neurosurgical units.

Summary

- Neurosurgery is limited by the availability of highly trained professionals and resources.
- Interpretation of scan images is highly vital for accurate diagnosis and institution of appropriate treatment, which can have significant impact on patient care and outcome.
- Currently, there are various methods of transmitting important scan images to experienced medical staff for accurate interpretation.
- MMS technology is a readily available, simple, and cost-effective method for the transmission of scan images.
- The use of MMS technology in emergency neurosurgery services has been effective in enhancing the confidence of neurosurgeons in clinical decision making, reducing the need for hospital call-back and improving patient care.

References

1. Apple SL, Schmidt JH (2000) Technique for neurosurgically relevant CT image transfers using inexpensive video digital technology. Surg Neurol 53:411–416
2. Archbold HA, Guha AR, Shyamsundar S, McBride SJ, Charlwood P, Wray R (2005) The use of multi-media messaging in the referral of musculoskeletal limb injuries to a tertiary trauma unit using: a 1-month evaluation. Injury 36(4):560–566
3. Bartlett JR, Neil-Dwyer G (1979) The role of computerized tomography in the care of the injured. Injury 11(2):144–147
4. Eljamel MS, Nixon T (1992) The use of a computer-based image link system to assist inter-hospital referrals. Br J Neurosurg 6:559–562
5. Eze N, Lo S, Bray D, Toma AG (2005) The use of camera mobile phone to assess emergency ENT radiological investigations. Clin Otolaryngol 30(3):230–233
6. Gentleman D, Jennett B (1981) Hazards of inter-hospital transfer of comatose head-injured patients. Lancet 8251:853–854
7. Glowacki M, Czernicki Z, Mierzejewski M (2002) The first system of image transmission and neurosurgical telecommunication in Poland. Neurol Neurochir Pol 36(2):363–369
8. Goh KY, Lam CK, Poon WS (1997) The impact of teleradiology on the inter-hospital transfer of neurosurgical patients. Br J Neurosurg 11(1):52–56
9. Gray WP, Somers J, Buckley TF (1998) Report of a national neurosurgical emergency teleconsulting system. Neurosurgery 42(1):103–107
10. Houkin K, Fukuhara S, Selladurai BM et al (1999) Telemedicine in neurosurgery using international digital telephone services between Japan and Malaysia: technical note. Neurol Med Chir (Tokyo) 39:773–778

11. Jithoo R, Govender PV, Corr P, Nathoo N (2003) Telemedicine and neurosurgery: experi-
    ence of a regional unit based in South Africa. J Telemed Telecare 9(2):63–66
12. Karasti H, Peponen J, Tervonen O, Kuutti K (1998) The teleradiology system and changes
    in work practices. Comput Methods Program Biomed 57:69–78
13. Lee T, Latham J, Kerr RS et al (1990) Effect of a new computed tomographic image
    transfer system on management of referrals to a regional neurosurgical service. Lancet
    336(8707):101–103
14. Ng WH, Wang E, Ng I (2007) Multimedia messaging service teleradiology in the provision
    of emergency neurosurgery services. Surg Neurol 67(4):338–341
15. Poca MA, Sahuquillo J, Domenech P et al (2004) Use of teleradiology in the evaluation and
    management of head-injured patients. Results of a pilot study of a link between a district
    general hospital and a neurosurgical referral center. Neurocirugia (Astur) 15(1):17–35
16. Poon WS, Goh KY (1998) The impact of teleradiology on the inter-hospital transfer of
    neurosurgical patients and their outcome. Hong Kong Med J 4(3):293–295
17. Stormo A, Sollid S, Stormer J, Ingebrigtsen T (2004) Neurosurgical teleconsultations in
    northern Norway. J Telemed Telecare 10(3):135–138
18. Walters KA (1993) Telephoned head injury referrals: the need to improve the quality of
    information provided. Arch Emerg Med 10:29–34
19. Wong HT, Poon WS, Jacobs P et al (2006) The comparative impact of video consultation
    on emergency neurosurgical referrals. Neurosurgery 59(3):607–613
20. Yamada M, Watarai H, Andou T, Sakai N (2003) Emergency image transfer system through
    a mobile telephone in Japan: technical note. Neurosurgery 52(4):968–986

9

Ultrasound Image Transmission via Camera Phones

Michael Blaivas

Abstract Ultrasound is a modern imaging technique, which delivers no radiation and does not require injection of any chemicals to enhance visualization. Unlike other imaging modalities, it can reach locations that are inaccessible to plain X-rays, computed tomography, and magnetic resonance imaging. Ultrasound image transmission through camera phones can be useful in scenarios like remote locations, disaster scenes, battlefields, cruise ships, ground and air ambulances, and expeditions. The most important requirement for transmitting ultrasound images and video via camera phones is access to a network on which the camera phone can transmit data.

9.1
Introduction

Ultrasound is a somewhat unique modality among modern imaging. Unlike most imaging modalities, it delivers no radiation and does not require injection of potentially nephrotoxic chemicals to enhance visualization. In addition, it is very mobile and even portable, with several units now being available, which can be held not only with one arm but even in the palm of the hand. The use of ultrasound by clinicians outside of radiology and obstetrics dates back more than two decades but has now been accepted widely and is spreading rapidly throughout the world [3, 9, 10, 14, 15, 17]. Unlike other imaging modalities, ultrasound has rapidly made its way to locations that are inaccessible to plain X-rays, computed tomography (CT), and magnetic resonance imaging (MRI) [4, 8, 11].

Another unique and important difference of ultrasound is the requirement for the operator to know a considerable amount regarding ultrasound use and image acquisition, in order to perform studies [13]. While the amount of training can be modest and extensive experience is not needed for focused ultrasound examinations, the modality is operator-dependent [1]. Thus, someone who has no experience at all may have difficulty performing the scan adequately.

In contrast, CT requires knowledge of the machine, but then it takes over once the patient is positioned and a program is selected. This is not yet possible with ultrasound, and the operator is required to obtain each image and make certain that it is interpretable when working in the conventional setting.

Logic and experience suggest that in the case of the ultrasound operator, he or she would also be able to interpret the image. This is frequently the case as in the instance when the ultrasound technologist may be vastly more experienced with image interpretation than the reader, for example, if the reader specializes in MRI of the head and rarely reads the results of ultrasound examinations. In the clinical setting, when clinicians perform and interpret their own ultrasound examinations simultaneously, the ability to acquire an image goes hand in hand with the ability to interpret it. However, many focused ultrasound applications, which may make a life and death difference or improve medical system efficiency, can be performed by personnel with limited training and experience; thus, review of the images or even video may be helpful. It is in these scenarios that transmission of ultrasound images and video via camera phones become revolutionary.

9.2
Potential Uses

There are a multitude of potential uses for ultrasound transmission over camera phones. The pattern that applies most broadly is a requirement for additional interpretation or delivery of illustrative images to a remote source. Types of scenarios likely to benefit are not limited to but include remote locations, disaster scenes, battlefields, cruise ships, ground and air ambulances, and expeditions. In general, there will be three types of applications for image transmission via a camera phone from any of these sites. The first is the transmission of an image, images, or video from the bedside of a patient who is being scanned by a relatively inexperienced provider, when it comes to ultrasound. The images will be transmitted in order to obtain aid in interpretation of the anatomy and potential abnormality seen. The second general use is to provide information to a receiving facility and visual evidence of an abnormality identified on ultrasound examination. Thus, an experienced ultrasound practitioner may send a video of blood noted in the abdomen of an injured train crash victim to a hospital capable of treating such trauma patients. The images or video illustrates the significance of the bleeding identified and aids in convincing the receiving facility of the validity of a diagnosis. The third is some mixture of the two, where an operator finds an abnormality that he or she is not familiar with and requires additional expertise that is not immediately available. If an abnormality is confirmed, it may lead to patient transfer to another facility for treatment.

In the case of major disasters, large numbers of casualties may have to be evaluated rapidly. Examples are train derailments, earthquakes, and terrorist acts [6, 7, 12]. In many cases, the first medical personnel on the scene will encounter a large percentage of blunt trauma victims and have limited resources. The main goal of ultrasound use is to evaluate dozens and perhaps even hundreds of blunt trauma victims to look for bleeding in the abdomen or perhaps signs of lung collapse in the thorax (Armenian quake) [18]. However, as the emergency medical technician starts scanning with ultrasound, she or he transmits images of the scans using a camera phone. This allowed the nearest trauma hospital to identify the first 16 victims, out of 95, who needed to be transported out right away and go to their facility for possible operative intervention. Most of the others would go to smaller nearby hospitals to have been treated for less life-threatening injuries. The battlefield setting will be quite similar (Fig. 9.1). Those found to have significant

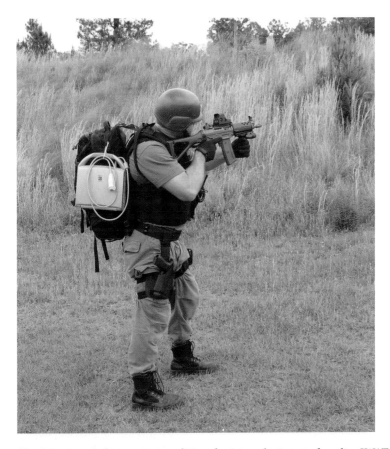

Fig. 9.1. A tactical emergency medicine physician who is part of a police SWAT team carries a compact ultrasound unit attached to his backpack. Shortly after this image was taken the machine was utilized to scan nine patients during a large-scale narcotic raid

injuries may be flown out to the forward hospital and others may be treated at the scene or in an aid station.

As cruising on ships becomes more and more popular, ships become larger and carry more passengers. Medical emergencies on cruise ships are not rare, and some may need to be evacuated [16]. This can include trauma as described above, but more likely it will mean other disease states such as ectopic or tubal pregnancies in female passengers and abdominal aortic aneurysms in older passengers. Many patients of different ages traveling on ships will be at risk of gallbladder complications, with stones leading to obstruction and gallbladders then becoming inflamed and infected. In many cases, such patients may require evacuation and surgery. There is a long list of other medical diseases that would benefit from ultrasound evaluation as well. A camera phone would be useful in transmitting images to a possible receiving hospital to help in interpretation and also to determine the need and urgency of patient evacuation. If a ship does not possess direct satellite linkage to its ultrasound machine, the camera phone may be used as a bridge to transmit images to the ship's wireless system or, if satellite-equipped, it may send the image directly to the ship, when out at sea.

Ground or air ambulances transporting patients over distances taking more than just a few minutes often not only have the time to reevaluate a patient en route but may also have to address changes in the patient's appearance or vital signs. For longer transport times that may range from 45 min to several hours, the patient may be examined several times. The discovery of a serious abnormality on ultrasound examination, such as blood in the abdomen or a collapsed lung, may be important information for the receiving facility. It may even lead to diversion of the ambulance to a different facility, which may be closer and ready to help treat the patient. Many ground and air transports occur within easy reach of established mobile-phone towers.

Another important use is in less densely populated portions of the globe such as rural areas or highly underserved areas, which can be found outside larger cities in Africa but may still be densely populated by Western standards. In either case, advanced and expensive imaging equipment may not be available and ultrasound may be the only feasible imaging approach. A portable ultrasound machine can be brought to the patient's bedside in a small village, farm, or ranch and images may be transmitted to a receiving facility via a camera phone. Identification of an abnormality that requires evacuation of the patient as opposed to something that can be treated locally can tremendously increase efficiency, when the cost of transporting a patient hundreds of miles may be very high and it may even be dangerous to do so.

A system utilizing camera phones to transmit ultrasound images can have a significant impact in clinical practice. With the continued spread of emergency ultrasound, real-time feedback on an abnormality and diagnosis can be provided easily by those more experienced in the field. Such consultation may not just deliver an image to a far-away reviewer but may also help reduce medical errors, by encouraging the use of emergency ultrasound, which has been shown to prevent unnecessary treatment, when a colleague sends an unclear finding to another colleague at home or at another institution [2]. Additionally, the novice user can be provided with real-time quality assurance from the director of clinical ultrasound and ongoing education if there exists any diagnostic uncertainty.

The camera mobile phone offers additional benefits. The camera phone can send pictures to several phones and e-mail addresses simultaneously. Therefore, the clinical department could have a quality assurance address to which images or videos are sent. A database would then be built simultaneously with the quality assurance process. This is advantageous, as some emergency ultrasound examinations may require follow-up evaluations at some point in the future.

The start-up costs for a system utilizing camera phones for ultrasound transmission are quite low. In fact, many first providers and other medical personnel who would be utilizing such a system may already privately own mobile phones that are ideal for use. Thus, an informal system could be set up almost immediately. However, a more formal system utilizing higher-resolution cameras and standard equipment should still cost less than $1,000 in most cases, and frequently much less. There may be additional communication charges for each video or picture sent, but this may also be included in an ongoing monthly maintenance cost. Image transfer is not instantaneous, but, when timed, studies showed them to take less than 2 min in most cases. Further, since medical data may be considered confidential, patient information is protected by the server in the same manner as is e-mail between personal computers. However, if this method of security for data transfer is not enough, patient names and personal information are easily left off the images and video.

9.3
Challenges

Multiple challenges exist to the idea of transmitting ultrasound images and video via camera phones. The first and foremost is having access to a network on which the camera phone can transmit data. This is actually a rapidly shrinking problem in much of the world. In industrialized countries, large mobile-phone networks exist, which can frequently be accessed by first providers and ambulance personnel. Even in less developed portions of the world where ground lines may be lacking, mobile-phone services are often easily available. For example, the cost and feasibility of laying ground lines in portions of India or Africa was prohibitive, while putting up a mobile-phone tower every several miles was possible. Even if a service is not available for the entire length between a small village clinic and a regional hospital, a mobile connection may be present in the village and may allow a camera phone to transmit ultrasound images to the receiving location.

Alternatively, the use of satellite mobile phones has the potential of providing a ready connection in almost any part of the world. This will require specialized equipment, which is typically more expensive and bulky. However, many satellite phones may be camera-equipped and can transmit still images and video. This technology is most likely to be applied during expeditions to remote locations such as jungle areas or mountains, the North Pole and the South Pole, and even Mount Everest.

A benefit of most modern mobile phones is the ability to obtain images through a camera and, in many cases, video (Fig. 9.2). Additionally, most are adapted to receive images and video from other camera phones, making it easy to send images from the source and have them reviewed at the receiving facility or anywhere the reviewer happens to be. An alternative is to send images via e-mail, and this may be especially convenient to do with short video clips showing portions of the examination. Physicians at the receiving facility, such as the emergency

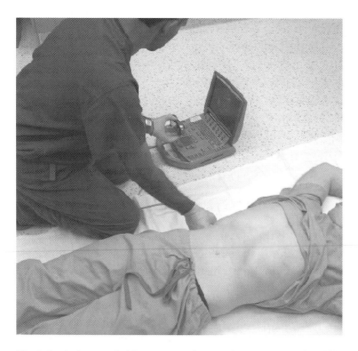

Fig. 9.2. A clinician holds a camera phone as he scans a simulated blunt trauma victim during a simulated disaster exercise. The camera phone records the images on the screen for a 30–60-s video covering the entire trauma examination. The video is then transmitted to several receivers 250 km away

physician in charge, can review the video or still images sent as e-mail attachments and replay and even manipulate the data repeatedly if needed. From here, the data can also be forwarded to other location, perhaps such as the operating room where a surgeon is now working, to let him/her know that more business is on its way. In fact, many camera phones with video capability could capture an entire-minute-long trauma ultrasound examination and then rapidly transmit it.

Image resolution and size are important issues to consider. Unlike a hazy and pixilated image of one's friend at a birthday party or the out-of-focus picture taken of a celebrity at a dark restaurant on a camera phone, a picture intended for medical interpretation has several requirements. The image or video must speak for itself. While you may be able to convince your friends that it was really a movie star among the shadows and pixels your camera phone captured, the medical image must be clear. The transmitted image of the ultrasound scan, or a video of the scan, must be easily readable by the receiver (Fig. 9.3).

If an ultrasound image is too grainy or hazy or too small it may be too difficult to read, but how do we decide what the limits are beyond which images are not useful? Currently, most mobile camera phones have a resolution of 640 × 480 pixels or better (Fig. 9.4). In fact, it is no longer uncommon to find standard cameras on mobile phones that have resolutions of 2 megapixels. Video recording on cameras has progressed rapidly as well, and many allow video to be recorded in near real time and then rapidly transmitted (Fig. 9.5).

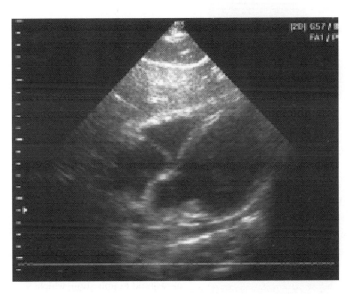

Fig. 9.3. A standard thermal ultrasound printout. It is considered to be of acceptable resolution and quality for ultrasound image transmission. In this case, the heart is showing at the *bottom* of the image, with all four chambers seen

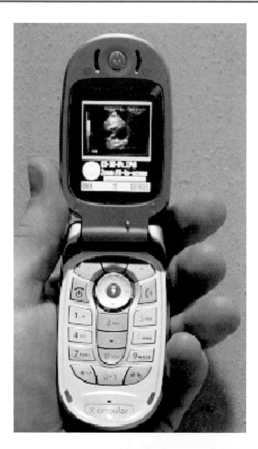

Fig. 9.4. The same image as shown in Fig. 9.3 has now been captured by a camera phone and transmitted 250 km from a disaster exercise. The image is smaller but can still be read

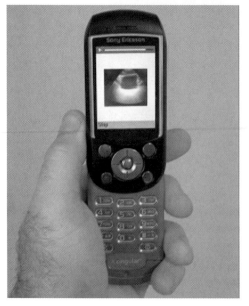

Fig. 9.5. A camera phone capable of capturing and receiving video. It has just finished playing a 45-s video showing a trauma abdominal ultrasound examination, which ended with a normal but full bladder. The images were obtained during a feasibility study 250 km away

Previous studies have suggested that the resolution required to make a diagnosis from a medical image can vary, depending on the type of image being interpreted. For instance, mammography requires higher resolution for diagnostic purposes than that needed for CT, which typically uses a 512×512 matrix at an 8-bit gray level. However, compared with analog images, 80% of viewers found digital images with resolution as low as 530×400 to be indistinguishable from the originals [19]. These digital images are the kinds that would be sent via a mobile phone equipped with a camera. A study evaluating images obtained by a mobile camera phone of CT and MRI scans showed that they were of sufficient quality for interpretation. In this particular study, the mobile-phone camera used had a display size of 31 mm $\times$ 30 mm and only 120×128 pixels resolution (110,000 pixels) [20]. This resolution is considerably less than what is available now on most of the basic mobile phones.

Another study that evaluated transmission of a wide variety of ultrasound images indicated that while images are not the same on a camera phone as a high-resolution thermal print, reviewers were still able to accurately interpret the images [5]. Researchers used an off-the-shelf camera phone that captured still images with a resolution of 640×480 pixels in color. The authors showed that there was no statistically significant difference in resolution, detail, and image quality scores between the high-resolution thermal prints and digital mobile camera phone images on a ten-point Likert scale. There were some drawbacks of the camera phone images, however. The reviewers were less confident in the interpretation of the image from a camera phone compared with the thermal prints. This obviously suggests that the two are not identical in quality. Agreement was good among reviewers for identification of important structures between image types, as well as among themselves. This study also identified another important drawback that may apply, especially to smaller mobile camera phones. This was the inability of reviewers to read most measurements, which appeared to be too small on the camera phone images. In most situations, however, the sender of the images could verbally relay measurements when discussing the case with a reviewer using a mobile phone.

A study conducted by us that is currently in print evaluated trauma ultrasound examination video transmission from a simulated disaster scene. The setting was a mass-casualty event simulated for a large training exercise occurring for a regional government. Selected casualties were brought to an emergency medical area, where rapid ultrasound trauma examinations were performed and recorded in real time on a mobile video camera phone. The images were then transmitted approximately 250 km away via a mobile phone and reviewed by three blinded reviewers. Even in the setting of rain and poor lighting conditions outside, chosen over the well-lit and dry areas available nearby to simulate a more adverse setting, the reviewers had high confidence in the video they viewed and felt that they could make a reliable diagnosis. Situations like this are occurring more and more frequently around the world, and although this one was staged as a large terrorist act it also doubled well as a natural disaster where many casualties were evaluated and treated at one time.

9.4
Image Transmission

A picture is worth a thousand words. If one picture can tell you all that, then a video is worth a million words. When a patient's life may hang in the balance, sometimes the more the information, the better it is. A problem that has plagued traditional imaging providers, who still read ultrasound images acquired by a technologist performing the scan but never scan the patient themselves, is that an ultrasound image is a two-dimensional slice through three-dimensional space and can miss everything just to one side of it or another. Many misdiagnoses have occurred this way. A video that covers an entire scan through an organ, or several organs, however, is less likely to lead to something being missed. Thus, a video is frequently preferred over still images, especially if the operator who is scanning with the ultrasound machine has very limited experience.

Transmission speed can be an important issue as well. One of the quoted studies listed the transmission speed as 14,000 bytes/s upload and 9,000 bytes/s download [5]. The authors noted few delays, however. What is interesting is the fact that many mobile-phone networks have tremendously faster download and upload speeds, sometimes several fold faster. Thus, as technology rapidly races ahead of us, these concerns become less and less significant on a monthly basis.

How many images should one send? Again, we are back to the one picture worth a thousand words versus a video worth a million words concept. The answer is to send as few images as possible, but these should still tell everything necessary. In the case of a blunt trauma victim with an abdomen full of blood it may be only one image, that of the liver and kidney separated by a thick stripe of black (fluid). In the case of a complicated finding in the pelvis of a patient with first trimester pain and bleeding, it may require multiple images or, best yet, a video showing a sweep through the pelvis in two orthogonal planes.

9.5
Conclusion

The potential use of camera phones for ultrasound image transmissionis significant and is growing on a regular basis, as more robust emergency systems are developed to respond to both natural and unnatural disasters. In addition, ultrasound remains the only medical imaging system that can be easily moved to the point of care, where the patient can be evaluated rapidly and critical decisions regarding transfer and treatment can be made.

Summary

- Ultrasound is a modern imaging technique, which delivers no radiation and does not require injection of any chemicals to enhance visualization.
- Unlike other imaging modalities, ultrasound can reach locations that are inaccessible to plain X-rays, CT, and MRI.
- Ultrasound image transmission via camera phones can be useful in scenarios like remote locations, disaster scenes, battlefields, cruise ships, ground and air ambulances, and expeditions.
- The most important requirement for transmitting ultrasound images and video via camera phones is access to a network on which the camera phone can transmit data.

References

1. American College of Emergency Physicians (2001) ACEP emergency ultrasound guidelines-2001. Ann Emerg Med 38:470–481
2. Blaivas M, DeBehnke D, Phelan MB (2000) Potential errors in the diagnosis of pericardial effusion on trauma ultrasound for penetrating injuries. Acad Emerg Med 7:1261–1266
3. Blaivas M, Lambert MJ, Harwood RC et al (2000) Lower-extremity Doppler for deep venous thrombosis – can emergency physicians be accurate and fast? Acad Emerg Med 7:120–126
4. Blaivas M, Kuhn W, Reynolds B, Brannam L (2005) Change in differential diagnosis and patient management with the use of portable ultrasound in a remote setting. Wilderness Environ Med 16:38–41
5. Blaivas M, Lyon M, Duggal S (2005) Ultrasound image transmission via camera phones for overreading. Am J Emerg Med 23:433–438
6. De Lorenzo RA, Augustine JJ (1996) Lessons in emergency evacuation from the Miamisburg train derailment. Prehosp Disaster Med 11:270–275
7. Gnauck KA, Nufer KE, LaValley JM, Crandall CS, Craig FW, Wilson-Ramirez GB (2007) Do pediatric and adult disaster victims differ? A descriptive analysis of clinical encounters from four natural disaster DMAT deployments. Prehosp Disaster Med 22:67–73
8. Huffer LL, Bauch TD, Furgerson JL, Bulgrin J, Boyd SY (2004) Feasibility of remote echocardiography with satellite transmission and real-time interpretation to support medical activities in the austere medical environment. J Am Soc Echocardiogr 17:670–674
9. Kirkpatrick AW, Jones JA, Sargsyan A et al (2007) Trauma sonography for use in microgravity. Aviat Space Environ Med 78:A38–A42
10. Lichtenstein DA, Menu Y (1995) A bedside ultrasound sign ruling out pneumothorax in the critically ill. Lung sliding. Chest 108:1345–1348

11. Lyon M, Blaivas M, Brannam L (2005) Use of emergency ultrasound in a rural ED with limited radiology services. Am J Emerg Med 23:212–214

12. Ma OJ, Norvell JG, Subramanian S (2007) Ultrasound applications in mass casualties and extreme environments. Crit Care Med 35:S275–S279

13. Moneta GL, Zierler RE, Zierler BK (2006) Training and credentialing in vascular laboratory diagnosis. Semin Vasc Surg 19:205–209

14. Neri L, Storti E, Lichtenstein D (2007) Toward an ultrasound curriculum for critical care medicine. Crit Care Med 35:S290–S304

15. Plummer D (1989) Principles of emergency ultrasound and echocardiography. Ann Emerg Med 18:1291–1297

16. Prina LD, Orzai UN, Weber RE (2001) Evaluation of emergency air evacuation of critically ill patients from cruise ships. J Travel Med 8:285–292

17. Rozycki GS, Ochsner MG, Jaffin JH, Champion HR (1993) Prospective evaluation of surgeons' use of ultrasound in the evaluation of trauma patients. J Trauma 34:516–526

18. Sarkisian AE, Khondkarian RA, Amirbekian NM, Bagdasarian NB, Khojayan RL, Oganesian YT (1991) Sonographic screening of mass casualties for abdominal and renal injuries following the 1988 Armenian earthquake. J Trauma 31:247–250

19. Schellingerhout D, Chew F, Mullins M, Gonzalez G (2002) Projected digital radiologic images for teaching. Acad Radiol 9:157–162

20. Yamada M, Watarai H, Andou T, Sakai N (2003) Emergency image transfer system through a mobile telephone in Japan: technical note. Neurosurgery 52:986–988

10

Clinical Teleradiology: Collaboration over the Web During Interventional Radiology Procedures

Lefteris G. Gortzis

Abstract Web-based collaborative clinical teleradiology can be looked upon as a set of services for quality assurance that enables expertise sharing and furthers health education opportunities. In particular, this set of services is a requisite of optimizing the final outcomes: structuring a common collaborative educational basis able to connect simultaneously distributed educators, students, and less experienced interventionists; eliminating the radiation dose constraints that arise from the continuous physical presence in the catheter laboratory of a high-volume center; and minimizing travel costs.

10.1
Background Information

Truly significant technological advances in the field of medicine are usually met with great acclaim, both in the medical community and in the public sector. Occasionally, though, changes occur, which become standard clinical practice easily and somewhat quietly.

Interventional radiology certainly does not fall exactly into that category. Coupled with and fuelled by parallel advances in computer technology, medical physics, and developments in endovascular catheter technology, interventional radiologists are innovating not only replacements for open surgeries, but entirely new therapies as well [19]. Based on such advantages, patients now reap the benefits of earlier diagnoses and less invasive treatment alternatives with lower morbidity and mortality.

In this clinical field, modern picture archiving and communication systems (PACS) and changes in infrastructure, together with faster communication networks and security in data and services exchange, are driving new service delivery models by applying clinical teleradiology [6].

There are many definitions of *clinical teleradiology*, but a reasonable working one defines it as the use of telecommunications to deliver real-time radiology services from one location to another for interpretation, consultation, and collaboration purposes [32].

Of all three, *collaboration* is probably the most critical, as it will contribute a great deal to spearheading the push for quality in real-world *interventional radiology procedure* (IRP) outcomes [12]. Collaboration is needed among organizations (e.g., local, national, international, etc.), professional groups (e.g., interventionists, physicists, technologists, etc.), and disciplines (e.g., interventionists, other clinical disciplines, etc.) to break down barriers, identify common goals, and pave the way for better-quality outcomes for patients [13, 30].

According to recent research [11], clinical teleradiology will benefit a lot from collaboration at a variety of levels as:

- IRP are often complex, and there is usually more than one objective to be achieved. For instance, in thrombolysis and inferior extremities cases (maximum IRP duration 3 h), surgeon collaboration is required.
- Several modern angiography units do not incorporate modern imaging facilities. One obvious solution would be to install advanced units. While this would partially solve the most important deficits, it would still not provide a satisfying outcome [16].
- There is lack of surveillance for reviewing and learning from possible methodological errors (diagnostic and therapeutic).
- Asynchronous scenarios that involve vascular surgeons at operating rooms, interventionists at catheter laboratories, and medical physicists at image-processing laboratories no longer satisfy modern requirements.

We should also point out that global experience has shown that collaboration can also play a vital role in the provision of learning contents. Synchronous and asynchronous Web-based modules can be used as adjuncts to traditional face-to-face education for supplementation and enrichment [29].

Hence, it is intriguing to consider which revolutionary changes have become adopted in routine IRP and what the next phase holds. In the following sections, a number of systems that promise to continue the technological revolution in these procedures will be examined.

10.2
Global Experience

Clinical teleradiology started as a point-to-point application and evolved into a mature set of services, based on several emerging business models [22]. Accordingly, many of the rules and practices that have governed traditional applications are being revised, and the lines that separated PACS from Web-browser environments are being blurred into a larger concept of collaborative multinode data management in the growing health-care enterprise.

Nowadays, clinical teleradiology is a broader concept, which has been driven in the health-care environments not by the shortage of interventionists but by the need for different departments, groups, or enterprises to expand essential services via a collaborative scheme improving the final IRP outcomes [22].

In the field of interventional radiology worldwide, significant heterogeneous systems are being directed toward providing collaborative services. In these systems, the most widely accepted scenario for the provision of collaboration patterns is typically that of several imaging modalities (e.g., computed tomography, magnetic resonance imaging, etc.) connected to a PACS archive and a number of reporting and reviewing nodes—there can be several onsite. According to this, Web clients (thin clients), can also view reports, images, and video—there can be several onsite and offsite—by being interconnected with the system interface.

Normally, such scenarios with a regular PACS would require expensive interface testing and configuration between multiple vendors running on a half-dozen computer systems. Unlike a traditional PACS, however, the Web-browser-based approaches provide medical facilities with the luxury of PACS without having a resident computer geek working full time.

A detailed literature study has shown that several systems are still oriented toward asynchronous collaboration between experts and other medical staff [4, 6, 18]. The applied collaboration pattern assumes communication via a central node where data concerning an IRP are stored. Usually, special toolbars allow specific operations to be performed on the images (brightness–contrast, zoom, distance measurement, and regions of interest, ROI, defining). Then the images could be accessed and evaluated remotely by experienced interventionists via any communication network.

Other systems use digital imaging and communications in medicine and/or health level 7 standards-based gateways and current robust suites of hardware options and software applications for data exchanging via any node with an Internet connection [18]. These systems facilitate electronic acquisition, viewing, communication/transmission, publishing, and storage of IRP data captured by numerous imaging modalities and devices and associated with a variety of medical subspecialties.

Many other systems support cooperative imaging diagnosis via a broadband multimedia teleradiology platform [10, 31]. These systems exploit the possibilities offered by asynchronous transfer mode technology or a public telecommunications integrated services digital network to support real-time teleconsultation services for medical imaging. On the other hand, Miyashita et al. [21] propose an ultrasound screening system which uses a scanner and a satellite telecommunication network. This single-screen unicast system appears to be a promising technique for those who live in rural communities, but it cannot support the current IRP collaboration requirements.

The multinode intraoperating IRP collaboration over the Web demands workflow-oriented services [1], bandwidth controlling [3], and a clinically accepted image compression [2, 36].

The collaboration patterns have recently been enhanced with modern technologies (scenarios, codec, hardware, etc.) that provide a standardized uniform platform for remote access from any connected node in a synchronous mode.

Progress in these technologies offers new possibilities of developing new collaborative services that are not subject to lack of real-time interactivity between an expert and other interventionists and sensitivity to computer network quality-of-service parameters. Utilizing these new technologies, Gortzis et al. [11] have developed a system, called NetAngio, which operates simultaneously in synchronous and asynchronous mode supporting "on the fly" multinode collaboration during real-world IRP, as shown in Fig. 10.1.

In this system, the authorized clinical collaborators (expert, interventionists, vascular surgeons, etc.) are able to participate, thus offering their contribution

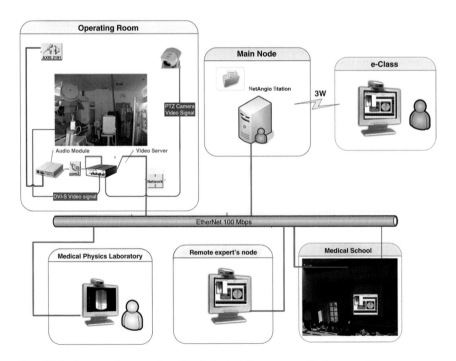

Fig. 10.1. System—Interventional Radiological Department, University of Patras

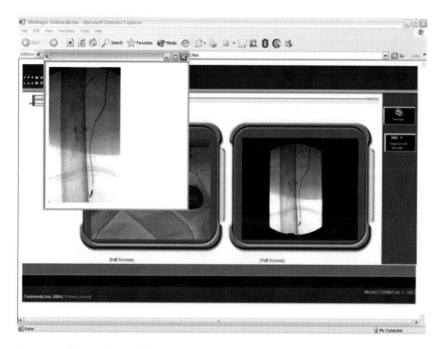

Fig. 10.2. Screen shot of the NetAngio system—Interventional Radiological department, University of Patras

and expertise through distance. Two dynamic film-based feeds (352×288) and the services' activation buttons are both contained in the main interface. The output angio-unit signal and the ceiling camera signal are both captured and displayed by the feeds, facilitating environment visual reconstruction.

Supported functions include (1) ceiling camera remote controlling (focus, position, and zoom), (2) multipoint conferencing, and (3) captured image forwarding. The image forwarding function is based on a "snap and forward" module able to post a suspect still-image to a remote medical physicist instantly. Following the data enhancement, a viewer—viewing Web module—grabs and displays them in a pop-up window on the main interface, as shown in Fig. 10.2.

Via a similar interface, at the same time, remote learners (students or less experienced interventional radiologists) are able to study the techniques performed and the collaborative consultation. The learner's access point, of course, based on a restricted interface designed just for educational objectives—ceiling camera controlling, is not supported.

We should emphasize that in this collaboration pattern, the role of the medical physicist is critical, as he/she is able to assist the remote mentor to propose better intraoperating planning treatment. In particular, he/she can collaborate with the mentor, locate the suspect ROI on received images, and enhance them by using locally installed biomedical imaging software system (Analyze version 5.0, Mayo Clinic) supporting the IRP.

10.3
Collaboration Patterns and E-learning

Electronic learning (e-learning) is an affordable and easy-to-use service that uses the Internet to give learners remote access to knowledge, immediate assessment of their understanding, and peer guidance as required. On this theoretical basis, more and more professionals are unraveling the modern e-learning as a new tool and attractive adjunct to the traditional teaching in medicine. Others think that we are currently witnessing another paradigm of permutation in medicine: a paradigm that sets these e-learning services and the new media in the center of interest. Nevertheless, all of them have accepted as a fact that we are entering a time when collaboration will also be an essential part of education in interventional radiology [26].

While previous collaboration learning systems included e-mail, computer networks, whiteboards, bulletin board modules, chat lines, and online presentation tools, current systems can include extensive mentoring networks, collaboration effectiveness indices, collaborative learning portals, chat networks, and freelance mentor exchange programs. An understanding, therefore, of these e-learning advances (synchronous and asynchronous) is an increasingly important part of modern interventional radiology, as there are already a number of promises associated with them.

10.3.1
E-learning in Synchronous Mode

The concept of synchronous or real-time learning, relative to other e-learning regimens, is quite new. The definition of what constitutes real-time e-learning still suffers from some ambiguities. It can be described as more than just a single instance of training and testing conveniently delivered. Real-time learning is about providing a service for collaborators, by connecting them to the strategy, tactics, policies, and procedures they need to accomplish increasingly complex tasks at the precise moment they need them. It is also about the method of delivery and the notion that IRP can be delivered visually to remote students at once.

On the basis of the scenarios highlighted above, we must consider that the next evolution in learning enterprise is a live, real-time IRP environment that provides collaborators with flow of information support as they perform their work.

In such collaborative scenarios, an experienced interventionist always acts as a mentor and presenter, providing opportunities for exploratory learning over the Web, based on various real-world IRP, independent of the time and place of the catheter laboratory.

Such learning displays the following characteristics:

- Ability of any learner or interventionist to lead discussions or present material
- Ability of the mentor, vascular surgeon, and students to share applications
- Availability of "breakout rooms" for small groups
- Availability of record and playback features for archiving and later review

10.3.2
E-learning in Asynchronous Mode

In addition to synchronous e-learning, there are opportunities for collaboration in asynchronous mode. A modern Web-based collaborative system can also operate in asynchronous mode to transfer, store, and retrieve digital medical videos and images for viewing at any place, and at any time. It can also integrate data from node to node, inside and outside an interventional radiology department, and ensure that video and related data are made available as needed, at the point of education, via video and audio streaming technologies.

Streaming is a technique of sending video and audio information in a compressed digital format. The Web tends to transfer deposited video and audio separated, but, in such services, there is the need for both of them to appear seamless at the viewing end [9]. For this reason, streaming is used widely, as it involves data digitization and transmission in a manner that appears almost smooth to the remote learner [9].

Such Web-based educational services can be accessed by multiple learners simultaneously, the only requirement being that they have an Internet connection and the appropriate hardware/software for viewing and listening installed on their node. The shared images are converted to either bitmap or Tagged Image File Format images by AGFA CS5000 software. The final resolution of the images may depend on the monitor and the video card installed in the computer used to display them. Usually, the visual data have reduced resolution and some details are significantly blurred, in order for typical software/hardware to be able to manage enough information to support e-learning.

Questions can also be posed on the part of the learner via e-mail. From the point of view of the audience collaborator, this is a very simple and widely available interface to use.

Summarizing, we can indicate that the basic difference between synchronous and asynchronous e-learning is that the latter does not provide interactivity, and comments online between mentor and learner cannot be exchanged. This makes asynchronous e-learning often difficult and less efficient.

10.4
Future Directions

The majority of the views mentioned in this chapter introduce a new notion of collaboration, which assumes that, with the current technological advantages, a team of multidisciplinary experts located in geographically distributed nodes is able to work in real-time manner upon the same IRP data, sharing access to them, and exchanging services via Web-browser-based modules. In that sense, the advantages elevate collaboration to a higher, more advanced state, enabling not only telediagnosis and teleconsultation but also a number of essential services.

From the technical point of view, the key challenge in future approaches is how to implement tools and online exchange service mechanisms efficiently in the context of constrained communication along with high demands of real-world IRP.

This new pattern of collaboration requires the construction of a highly interactive, collaborative Web environment, which should provide abstraction of a session (i.e., a group of objects associated with some common communication methods), and support full-duplex multipoint communication between an arbitrary number of connected nodes.

Additional issues will also possibly arise, as the sharing node community usually has different attributes (the number and types of collaborators, the types of tasks, the duration and scale of the interaction, and the resources shared).

Collaborative IRP over the Web is more than simple image exchange facilities; it can involve direct access to software, content, data sensors, and other resources. Such resource sharing is conditional, as each collaborator will make certain resources available within the constraints of time, location, and purpose. The sharing relations may vary over time in terms of shared resources, nature of access, and types of collaborators. The ability to delegate authority and privilege is also a complex task, as the same resource may be used in different ways, depending on the restrictions imposed on the sharing and the goals of sharing.

The next phase of the digital revolution in clinical teleradiology will take place through the dissemination of powerful handheld computers [24, 25]. Handheld computers are no longer considered simple electronic notebooks. They have many features (Wi-Fi adapters, high-quality imaging cards, database programs, and digital media) that make them an ideal unit. These improvements in display characteristics and wireless networking capabilities provide a mobile node for real-time collaboration.

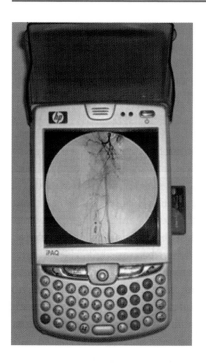

Fig. 10.3. Screen shot of the 4-bit (16-level) gray-scale display HP6515 with an SDIO wireless LAN card, NetAngio system

With the introduction of handheld computers into the IRP, some of the previous obstacles regarding place of work may be overcome. The most practical and cost-effective method to use a handheld computer will be to provide convenient access within an integrated scenario at the point where the IRP is taking place. This concept, known as "point-of-service" delivery is where the handheld computer is likely to establish itself as a clinical unit. Despite their small screen size (and font size) and the absence of a traditional keyboard, handheld computers may realize most of their use in the real-time review of clinical data and workflow management during a collaborative IRP, as shown in Fig. 10.3.

The next phase of the digital revolution in clinical teleradiology will also take place through multicast communication technologies. These technologies will have great advantages in this area, because they provide [8, 35] (1) interoperability, (2) stability and dependability, (3) guaranteed bit rate, and (4) optimal performance, based on the user datagram protocol.

In the future, the multicast systems will utilize effectively the appropriate number of video feeds, in order to reconstruct visually and in detail the remote catheter laboratory, while they will provide the collaborators with a number of value-added interactive functions (pointers, file transfer, whiteboard, etc.). Active involvement with such systems will enable the interventionists with medium-level expertise to operate independently, reducing expert workload and out-of-limits radiation exposure, optimizing substantially the overall departmental clinical practice [11].

Data compression certainly plays an important role in supporting multicast services under complex collaboration patterns effectively. For instance, compressed video should be useful to the remote interventionist, not necessarily better or worse than direct examination [33], while shared video volume should be according to the available communication bandwidth. The future system should employ low bit rate video compressions based on wavelet transform schemes, e.g., concepts of partition, aggregation, and conditional coding (PACC) [20]. The PACC codec is a possible solution to supporting multiple collaborative services via a hybrid network (e.g., terrestrial satellite), since it does not perform complex motion estimations and compensations. Moreover, it does not lose diagnostic content, succeeding in reduction of blocking artifacts better than others (e.g., the DCT-based H.263) [5, 7, 15, 23, 34].

Although the previous collaborative systems have been in use, most of them are still evolving, as there are a number of technical and regulatory issues associated with them, which system designers should take into consideration until they opt for a generally accepted model.

Finally, we should note that although technological advantages give healthcare delivery the potential to improve patient care, serious concerns are raised as to who should get access to collaborative sessions and how they should be protected.

Legal considerations are important in the evolving Web-based services and clinical teleradiology. Like all telemedicine services, teleradiology applications face regulatory and medical–legal concerns, particularly with regard to licensing, liability, confidentiality, security of information, and retention of records. The future key activities in security should include (1) monitoring and adjusting to the changing laws, regulations, and standards, (2) developing, implementing, and continuously updating security policies and procedure practices, and (3) institutionalizing responsibility for information security.

Considering the aforementioned, we can conclude that Web-based collaborative services provide treatment options not previously available for interventional radiology, but several issues can still be considered as possible disadvantages [28]. The lack of clear reimbursement of these services usually also hinders their widespread application [17].

We believe that the socioeconomic effects of the collaborative systems will become tangible only when these supported services become a mature part of interventional radiology. Only at that point will managers and decision makers gather clear evidence of the benefits of such systems and finally accept clinical teleradiology as a major requirement of routine health-care practice [14, 27].

Summary

Web-based collaborative clinical teleradiology can be looked upon as a set of services for quality assurance that enables expertise sharing and furthers health education opportunities.

In particular, this set of services is a requisite of:

- Optimizing the final outcomes
- Structuring a common collaborative educational basis able to connect simultaneously distributed educators, students, and less experienced interventionists
- Eliminating the radiation dose constraints that arise from the continuous physical presence in the catheter laboratory of a high-volume center
- Minimizing travel costs

References

1. Bashshur R, Shannon G, Sapci H (2005) Telemedicine evaluation. Telemed J E-Health 11(3):296–316
2. Begg L, Chan FY, Edie G, Hockey R, Wootton R (2001) Minimum acceptable standards for digital compression of a fetal ultrasound video-clip. J Telemed Telecare 7(Suppl 2):88–90
3. Bergh B, Schlaefke A, Pietsch M, Garcia I, Vogl TJ (2003) Evaluation of a "no-cost" Internet technology-based system for teleradiology and co-operative work. Eur Radiol 13(2): 425–434
4. Boehm T, Handgraetinger O, Link J et al (2004) Evaluation of radiological workstations and web-browser-based image distribution clients for a PACS project in hands-on workshops. Eur Radiol 14(5):908–914
5. Brennecke R, Burgel U, Rippin G, Post F, Rupprecht HJ, Meyer J (2001) Comparison of image compression viability for lossy and lossless JPEG and wavelet data reduction in coronary angiography. Int J Cardiovasc Imaging 17(1):1–12
6. Caffery L, Manthey K (2004) Implementation of a web-based teleradiology management system. J Telemed Telecare 10(Suppl 1):22–25
7. Cooper JB, Barron D, Blum R, et al (2000) Video teleconferencing with realistic simulation for medical education. J Clin Anesth 12(3):256–261
8. Duffy JR, Werven GW, Aronson AE (1997) Telemedicine and the diagnosis of speech and language disorders. Mayo Clin Proc 72(12):1116–1122
9. Garrison W (2001) Video streaming into the mainstream. J Audiovis Media Med 24(4):174–178
10. Gomez EJ, Caballero PJ, Malpica N, Del Pozo F (2001) Optimisation and evaluation of an asynchronous transfer mode teleradiology co-operative system: the experience of the emerald and the bonaparte projects. Comput Methods Prog Biomed 64(3): 201–214
11. Gortzis L, Karnabatidis D, Siablis D, Nikiforidis G (2006) Clinical-oriented collaborative work over web during interventional radiological procedures. Telemed E-Health 12(4):448–456

12. Gortzis GL, Papadopoulos H, Roelofs AT et al (2007) Collaborative work during interventional radiological procedures based on a multicast satellite-terrestrial network. IEEE Trans Inf Technol Biomed 11(5):597–599

13. Green RM (2000) Collaboration between vascular surgeons and interventional radiologists: reflections after two years. J Vasc Surg 31(4):826–830

14. Hu PJ, Chau PYK, Liu Sheng OR, Yan Tam K (1999) Examining the technology acceptance model using physician acceptance of telemedicine technology. J Manage Inform Syst 91–112

15. Itu-T Rec. H-261, (1993) "Video CODEC for Audiovisual services at p X 64 kbit/s"

16. Jacob AL, Regazzoni P, Steinbrich W, Messmer P (2000) The multifunctional therapy room of the future: image guidance, interdisciplinarity, integration and impact on patient pathways. Eur Radiol 10(11):1763–1739

17. Lamonte MP, Bahouth MN, Hu P et al (2003) Telemedicine for acute stroke: triumphs and pitfalls. Stroke 34(3):725–728

18. Luccichenti G, Ngo Dinh N, Cademartiri F, Evangelisti G, Paolillo A, Bastianello S (2004) Teleradiology system accessible through a common web browser. Radiol Med (Torino) 108(5–6);542–548

19. Luney SR (2002) Interventional radiology. Curr Opin Anaesthesiol 15(4):449–454

20. Marpe D, Cycon H (1999) Very low bit-rate video coding using wavelet-based techniques. IEEE Trans Circuits Syst Video Technol 9(1):85–94

21. Miyashita T, Takizawa M, Nakai K et al (2003) Realtime ultrasound screening by satellite telecommunication. J Telemed Telecare 9(Suppl 1):S60–S61

22. Mun SK, Tohme WG, Platenberg RC, Choi I (2005) Teleradiology and emerging business models. J Telemed Telecare 11(6):271–275

23. Munteanu A, Cornelis J, Cristea P (1999) Wavelet-based lossless compression of coronary angiographic images. IEEE Trans Med Imaging 18(3):272–281

24. Nishino M, Busch JM, Wei J, Barbaras L, Yam CS, Hatabu H (2004) Use of personal digital assistants in diagnostic radiology resident education. Acad Radiol 11(10):1153–1158

25. Raman B, Raman R, Raman L, Beaulieu CF (2004) Radiology on handheld devices: image display, manipulation, and PACS integration issues. Radiographics 24(1):299–310

26. Scarsbrook AF, Graham RN, Perriss RW (2006) Radiology education: a glimpse into the future. Clin Radiol 61(8):640–648

27. Sheng OR, Hu PJ, Chau PY et al (1998) A survey of physicians' acceptance of telemedicine. J Telemed Telecare 4(Suppl 1):100–102

28. Tyrer HW, Wiedemeier PD, Cattlet RW (2001) Rural telemedicine: satellites and fiber optics. Biomed Sci Instrum 37:417–422

29. Varga-Atkins T, Cooper H (2005) Developing e-learning for interprofessional education. J Telemed Telecare 11(Suppl 1):102–104

30. Verdun FR, Aroua A, Trueb PR, Vock P, Valley JF (2005) Diagnostic and interventional radiology: a strategy to introduce reference dose level taking into account the national practice. Radiat Prot Dosimetry 114(1–3):188–191

31. Welz R, Ligier Y, Ratib O (1995) Design of a cooperative teleradiology system. Telemed J 1(3):195–201

32. Wright R, Loughrey C (1995) Teleradiology. BMJ 310(6991):1392–1393

33. Yagi Y, Gilbertson JR (2005) Digital imaging in pathology: the case for standardization. J Telemed Telecare 11(3):109–116

34. Yamakawa T, Toyabe S, Cao P, Akazawa K (2004) Web-based delivery of medical multimedia contents using an MPEG-4 system. Comput Methods Prog Biomed 75(3):259–264

35. Yamauchi K, Ikeda M, Ota Y et al (2000) Evaluation of the space collaboration system: its history, image quality and effectiveness for joint case conference. Nagoya J Med Sci 63(1–2):19–24
36. Zhang Y, Pham BT, Eckstein MP (2005) Task-based model/human observer evaluation of SPIHT wavelet compression with human visual system-based quantization. Acad Radiol 12(3):324–336

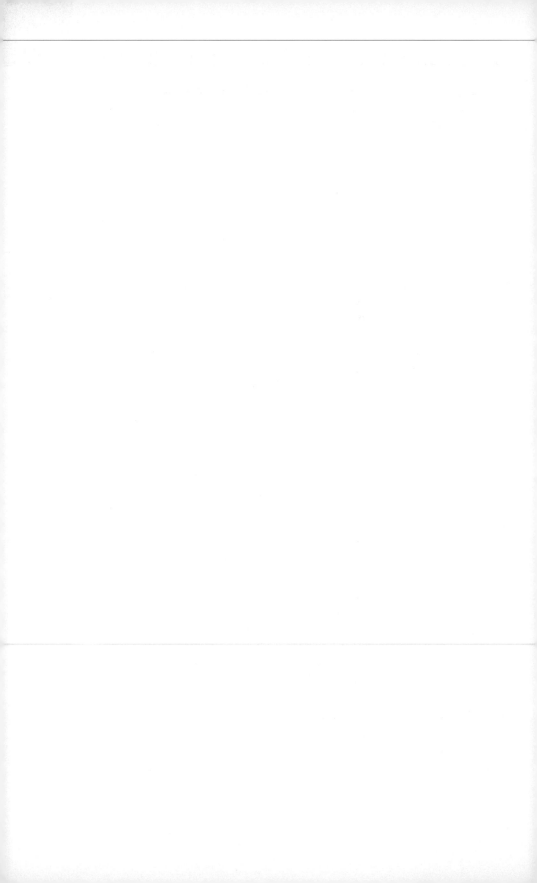

11

Teleplanning in Image-Guided Dental Implantology

Kurt Schicho and Rolf Ewers

Abstract Using the "augmented reality" principle, one can perceive real structures and additional computer-generated information synchronously, enabling a more comprehensive judgment of the situation almost in real time. Dental implantology is a typical example of preoperative teleplanning. "Telenavigation client" software that has been successfully tested in computer-assisted dental implantology allows real-time transmission of data from the position-tracking unit of a navigation system to an unlimited number of computers connected to the Internet.

11.1
Introduction

11.1.1
The Main Idea

The increasing clinical relevance of computer-assisted navigation technology in several fields of medicine since the early 1990s also promoted new perspectives in telemedicine [2–4]. When we define telemedicine as "any transmission of medical information by means of telecommunication technology," the central idea characterizing the specific advantages of telemedicine in combination with image-guided surgery becomes clear: Any "digital" content, i.e., digital images from imaging modalities (most frequently computed tomography, CT, and magnetic resonance imaging) as well as navigation data (e.g., intraoperative coordinates of surgical instruments relative to preplanned pathways and target points at the patient, implant positions, etc.), can be transferred without any loss of information (Fig. 11.1). This means that remote experts can be involved in surgical interventions or preoperative planning sessions while being supplied with information identical to that which the "local" staff receives. Furthermore, the same infrastructure can be utilized for continuous medical training and education, allowing the students to participate always in "real" cases independently of their geographic location.

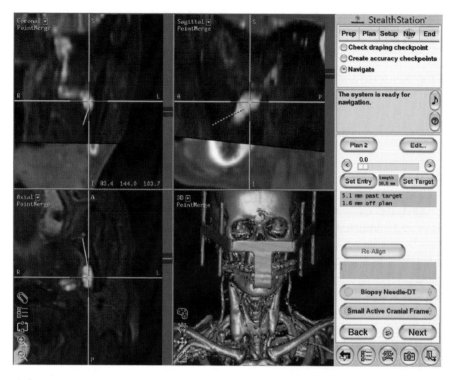

Fig. 11.1. Intraoperative screen of a navigation-supported biopsy in the facial area. In order to visualize hard and soft tissues, computed tomography (CT) and magnetic resonance imaging images were merged. The two- and three-dimensional images of the patient's "real" anatomy are superimposed with additional computer-generated information, in this example the *green line* representing the entry point and the trajectory for the biopsy needle. The digital images as well as the data for the exact navigational information (coordinates) can be transmitted via telecommunication without any loss of information. Furthermore, remote experts can directly be involved in the operation, using simple remote-control software for the navigation computer. This concept eliminates sources of errors due to misunderstandings like in spoken or written communication and therefore clearly surpasses the "old ways of telecommunication"

11.1.2
The Augmented Reality Principle

The approach presented above is based on the so-called augmented reality principle. In contrast to "virtual reality," which stands for completely computer generated information content (as known from computer games or flight simulators), augmented reality expands the "real world" (i.e., the actual view onto the anatomical structures or the operating room site, etc.) by means of the integration of additional computer-generated information. This computer-generated information is usually computer graphics illustrating surgical pathways, implant positions, or target structures inside the patient's tissue. They are superimposed with the surgeon's original view and therefore build a kind of "augmented world." Real structures and additional computer-generated information can be perceived synchronously, enabling a more comprehensive judgment of the situation almost in real time. For the technical realization of this principle, head-mounted displays have proven to be advantageous and to meet the surgeons' requirements better than common computer displays [5].

11.1.3
Computer-Assisted Dental Implantology and Telecommunication

Although the main principle of teleconsultation in computer-assisted surgery is usually the same in numerous applications, in this chapter we

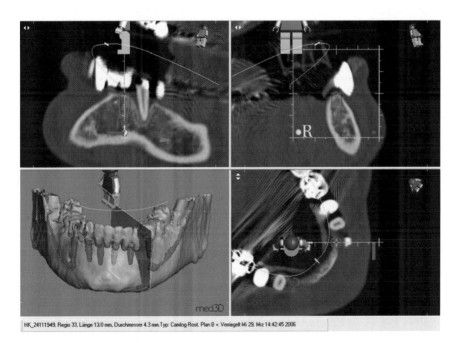

Fig. 11.2. Preoperative planning in computer-assisted dental implantology. On the basis of CT data, which have been transferred via the Internet, remote experts in a specialized center plan the positions and orientations of the implants in two- and three-dimensional views. The plan is returned online to the operating room (in cases where intraoperative navigation is applied), or it is used to provide the information for the production of surgical templates with rapid prototyping techniques. This example shows the software by Med3D (Med3D, Heidelberg, Germany); in the *lower-left* part of the screen, radio-opaque teeth on a temporary prosthesis are shown. The implants are aligned according to the axis of these temporary teeth ("backward planning with crown down implant positions")

focus on the specific tasks in dental implantology, because in this discipline we find intensive research and development activities and rapid technical progress [1].

For all the different concepts to supply patients with dental implants (e.g., common surgical drilling templates, intraoperative navigation, templates manufactured with rapid prototyping, etc.), CT data are the mandatory base for well-founded preoperative treatment planning. This CT data set can easily be transmitted from the radiologist to an experienced implant planning center, either on CD-ROMs via "snail-mail" or via the Internet (e.g., using the file transfer protocol). In such a center, the experts use special software that allows for comprehensive evaluation of the anatomical situation, in order to accomplish planning that optimizes the implantological restoration considering the available bone as well as all prosthetic, aesthetical, and functional aspects. This is a complex process that requires a high level of experience and routine. The computer-based plan is a file that can be returned to the surgeon online. In this step, all standards in security and integrity of the data have to be considered thoroughly, including national and international legislation. For the insertion of the implant, supported by either intraoperative navigation or template-based methods (e.g., manufactured with rapid-prototyping techniques), surgical skills are of course mandatory, but there is usually no additional advice from remote specialists. Therefore, dental implantology is a typical example for preoperative teleplanning. Live transmissions of the surgical intervention are usually only performed for education purposes, e.g., in the course of lectures.

11.1.4
Perspective: Surgical Training by Means of a Telenavigation Client

An innovation that has been successfully tested in computer-assisted dental implantology (but that is not at all limited to this specific application) is the so-called telenavigation client, developed by the Karl Landsteiner Institute for Biotelematics Vienna (Director Michael Truppe). This software allows real-time transmission of data from the position-tracking unit of a navigation system to an unlimited number of "clients," i.e., computers that are connected to the Internet. Before the beginning of an operation, CT data of the (anonymized) patient are downloaded to these clients. During the operation, each client computer acts as an independent navigation system; therefore, the user can arbitrarily select two- and three-dimensional views and cutting planes. Consequently, he/she can de facto participate in the operation without affecting the performance of the navigation computer in the operating room. The principle of the telenavigation client is illustrated in Fig. 11.3.

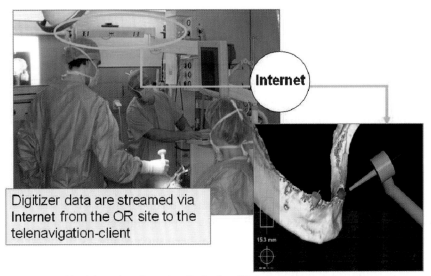

Karl Landsteiner Institute for Biotelematics, Vienna

a

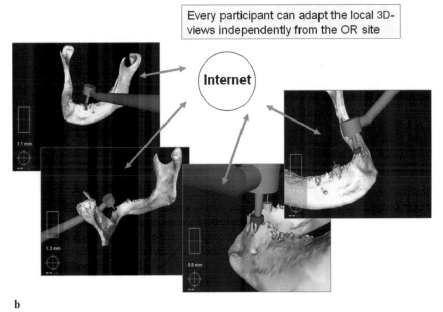

b

Fig. 11.3. Telenavigation client, developed by the Karl Landsteiner Institute for Biotelematics Vienna (Director Michael Truppe). During surgery real-time data (coordinates) from the position-tracking unit of the navigation system are **a** streamed via the Internet and **b** received by the client computers. At the client computers, which are independent navigation systems, the operation can be observed without affecting the performance of the computer at the operation site. *OR* operating room

Summary

- Telemedicine is the transmission of medical information by means of telecommunication technology.
- The advantages of telemedicine in combination with image-guided surgery are that digital images from imaging modalities can be transferred without any loss of information. So remote experts can be involved in surgical interventions or preoperative planning sessions. Furthermore, the same infrastructure can be utilized for continuous medical training and education.
- With use of the "augmented reality" principle, real structures and additional computer-generated information can be perceived synchronously, enabling a more comprehensive judgment of the situation almost in real time.
- Dental implantology is a typical example of preoperative teleplanning.
- "Telenavigation client" software that has been successfully tested in computer-assisted dental implantology allows real-time transmission of data from the position-tracking unit of a navigation system to an unlimited number of computers connected to the Internet.

References

1. Ewers R, Schicho K, Seemann R, Reichwein A, Figl M, Wagner A (2004) Computer aided navigation in dental implantology: 7 years of clinical experience. J Oral Maxillofac Surg 62:329–334
2. Ewers R, Schicho K, Undt G, Seemann R, Truppe M, Wagner A (2005) Seven years of clinical experience with teleconsultation in craniomaxillofacial surgery. J Oral Maxillofac Surg 63:1447–1454
3. Ewers R, Schicho K, Wanschitz F, Truppe M, Seemann R, Wagner A (2005) Basic research and 12 years of clinical experience in computer assisted navigation technology: a review. Int J Oral Maxillofac Surg 34:1–8
4. Wagner A, Undt G, Schicho K et al (2002) Interactive stereotaxic teleassistance of remote experts during arthroscopic procedures. Arthroscopy 18:1034–1039
5. Wanschitz F, Birkfellner W, Figl M et al (2002) Computer-enhanced stereoscopic vision in a head-mounted display for oral implant surgery. Clin Oral Implants Res 13:610–616

12

Web-Based Medical System for Managing and Processing Gynecological–Obstetrical–Radiological Data

George K. Matsopoulos, Pantelis A. Asvestas, Kostantinos K. Delibasis, Nikolaos A. Mouravliansky, and Vassilios Kouloulias

Abstract A Web-based teleradiology system, called MITIS, is presented for the management and processing of obstetrical, gynecological, and radiological medical data. The system records all the necessary medical information in terms of patient data, examinations, and operations and provides the user-expert with advanced image-processing tools for the manipulation, processing, and storage of ultrasonic and mammographic images. The system can be installed in a hospital's local area-network, where it can access picture archiving and communication system servers (if available), or any other server within the radiology department, for image archiving and retrieval, based on the DICOM 3.0 protocol over transmission control protocol/Internet protocol, and also it is accessible to external physicians via the hospital's Internet connection. The teleradiology system is composed as a set of independent Web modules and a Win32 application for mammographic image processing and evaluation.

12.1
Introduction

Teleradiology is the electronic transmission of a radiographic image from one geographical location to another for the purpose of interpretation and consultation. The development of medical digital imaging systems in conjunction with the improved capacity of the World Wide Web and the speed of transmission of large quantities of medical data have permitted a wider use of teleradiology, according to which all information and applications are stored in a locally centralized location and can be distributed over a network in several clients. The use of a standardized communication platform resulted in the development of various Web-based medical systems, which offer mainly new teleradiology services for a number of different medical cases [2].

In particular, teleradiology systems have been developed over the past few years, based on the Internet and the ubiquity of the Web browser. A complete and secure Internet-based teleradiology system, called JReads, has been developed for viewing medical images consisting of a Java applet at the front end, Java servlets and COBRA objects in the middle tier, and relational databases and image file servers at the back end [9]. In [17], a system was introduced using Web technologies and hypertext transfer protocol communication protocols for remotely processing ultrasonic images by using the angle-independent Doppler color image algorithm and by providing several image measurements through various Internet tools. Furthermore, another system was also introduced in [12], providing teleradiology services for radiotherapy treatment planning, whereas in [5], another teleradiology system, called KAMERIN, was reported for supporting cooperative work and remote image analysis of radiological data for ISDN-based telecommunication.

The implementation of the aforementioned teleradiology systems was based on the acceptance of a standard medical image communication protocol, known as digital imaging and communications in medicine (DICOM) [8], as well as on the development of picture archiving and communication systems (PACS) for handling and storing the image data generated by various medical modalities [3]. These Web-based systems involve medical experts from radiology departments. On the other hand, there is a strong need for incorporating experts from other departments and/or hospitals through such systems, such as experts from the obstetrics and gynecology departments. Of the references listed in this chapter, only a few research works have focused on the use of the Internet technology for obstetrical and gynecological purposes [4, 11].

In this chapter, we present a complete and secure Web-based system, called MITIS, for the management and processing of obstetrical, gynecological, and radiological medical data. The teleradiology system presented is a set of independent modules, connected with each other and fully compatible with the Web, thus providing flexibility and extensibility. It records all the necessary information related to patients' examination, operation, and any other gynecological data related to pregnancy and labor. It also incorporates computer graphics algorithms and advanced digital image-processing techniques for manipulating various medical images, including ultrasonic and mammographic data. An advantage of the system is the provision to the medical experts of a unified patient management mechanism, either in the hospital or outside. Furthermore, it offers cooperation of medical specialists from different medical departments, such as the obstetrics–gynecology department and the radiology department, either within the hospital and/or between hospitals or private offices, toward the monitoring of the progression of a disease and the establishment of a therapeutic scheme.

12.2
System Structure

12.2.1
General System Structure

Figure 12.1 shows the functional structure of the proposed teleradiology system. The system is a Web-based medical information system based on a three-tier client–server architecture and designed to provide mainly radiologists and gynecologists with unified patient management capabilities, either internally in the hospital or externally at a private office. According to Fig. 12.1, the system's server is originally installed in a hospital, and, via an Internet connection, it is accessible to other external physicians. On the server side, the system, via the local-area network (LAN) of the hospital, can access the

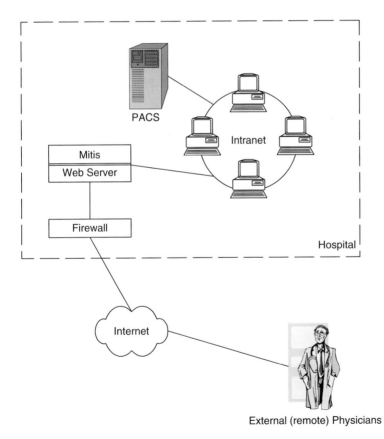

External (remote) Physicians

Fig. 12.1. General system structure. *PACS* picture archiving and communication system

hospital's PACS servers (if available), or any other server within the radiology department for image archiving and retrieval, based on the DICOM 3.0 protocol, over transmission control protocol/Internet protocol. External physicians access the system via the Internet, mostly via asymmetric digital subscriber line (ADSL) connections. These external physicians can be located in the same city, rural villages, or islands, and they can share the same patient information with the hospital. Thus, the system presented can serve two roles: (1) a patient medical record management system and (2) a system supporting teleradiology sessions of either different examinations and operations or remote medical image processing.

12.2.2
System Architecture

Figure 12.2 depicts the overall system architecture, which follows the three-tier model: hypertext markup language pages with client-site Java scripts and extensible markup language (XML) data islands at the front end, Internet server application programming interface (ISAPI) extensions (data link layers, DLLs) combined with Microsoft active server pages (ASP) in the middle tier, and a relational database management system with available ActiveX data object (ADO) drivers (Microsoft Structured Query Language Server 2000 preferable) at the back end. The system operates under Microsoft Windows NT/Internet information services (IIS) 4.0 or 2000/IIS 5.0 or newer platforms.

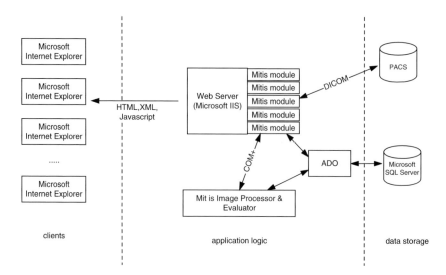

Fig. 12.2. Overall system architecture

The system was designed by making use of existing advanced Internet technologies and tools. Since one of the main requirements of the system was the compatibility with Web technologies, alternative scenarios of existing technologies along with combination with other supporting tools were initially evaluated. Table 12.1 depicts the technological scenarios, as well as criteria and scoring, available during the system's development period. From those criteria, the integration with other technologies refers to the integration with Windows NT and Windows 95 and up (Win32) application programming interface (API) services, while the development productivity is a combination of the level of expertise of the development team and the availability and cost of the development tools.

According to Table 12.1, the first solution of Microsoft ASP, connected with a database through ADOs, supports component object model (COM) technologies, but it has medium performance and development productivity. The PHP hypertext preprocessor, connected with a database through open database connectivity (ODBC), has the same disadvantages as ASP and furthermore limited integration with the operating system and external services. The ISAPI extensions with middle-tier common object request broker architecture, using AT&T's omni as the object request broker (ORB), have the disadvantage of low development productivity owing to the minimal support by rapid application development software tools such as Microsoft Visual Basic, Delphi, etc. The replacement of the ORB omni with a commercial product from Borland, such as VisiBroker, may offer a significant improvement in development productivity, with the disadvantage of a high deployment cost. The implementation of the client-side ActiveX, even though it increases the performance of the system, increases the bandwidth requirements considerably owing to higher network traffic, requires more computational power from the client (thick client), and is exposed to higher security threats (distribution and installation of ActiveX components only). The option of using Java applets/Java beans components to develop such a system as proposed was seriously considered for the particular application, but it was finally rejected owing to the higher level of expertise of the development team with the Win32 application and the better integration capabilities of the latter with Win32 API services. For similar reasons, the Java servlets/Java server pages were also excluded. The Microsoft.NET platform is a very powerful solution, but it was not fully available at the time of the development of the proposed system. For all the aforementioned reasons, the system was finally based on a mixture of the ISAPI extensions (DLLs) and ASP. This technology, made available by Borland, was initially developed for Delphi, and it is named Websnap.

The system is composed of a set of independent Web modules (ISAPI server extension DLLs) and a Win32 application (COM+ server) for mammographic

Table 12.1. Comparison of Web technologies for the development of the Teleradiology system presented in terms of specific criteria (the data refer to the period of the system's development)

Criteria	ASP	PHP	World Wide Web techniques					
			ISAPI extensions with ASP	ISAPI extensions with COBRA	Client side ActiveX	Java applets/ Java beans	Java servlets/JSP	Microsoft .NET
Performance	Medium	Medium	High	High	High	High	Medium	Medium
Integration with other technologies	High	Low	High	Medium	High	Medium	Medium	High
Development productivity	Medium	Medium	High	Low	High	Medium	Medium	Medium
Connectivity with databases	High	High	High	Medium	Medium	High	High	High
Security threats	Low	Medium	Low	Medium	High	Low	Low	Low
Bandwidth requirements	Low	Low	Low	Low	High	Medium	Low	Low
Deployment cost	Low	Low	Low	High	Low	High	Low	Low

ASP Active server pages, *PHP* Hypertext preprocessor, *ISAPI* Internet server application programming interface, *CORBA* Common object request broker architecture, *JSP* Java server pages

image processing and evaluation. The following modules have been developed and incorporated within the system:

- *Basic control module*: This module controls the user authentication, the display of persistent session information, the construction of the menu, and the system's login page. The module is declared in a simple XML file, which can easily be edited with a text editor. Also, in this module, an electronic scheduling tool is incorporated to manage all patient examinations. Furthermore, all the predefined parameters related to various medical examinations and operational findings, imported prior to the system, are configured through this module.

- *General data module*: This module supports all patients' general data, including past medical history (individual and hereditary), habits, allergies, drugs, etc. The patient's medical history data as well as the diagnostic data are coded according to the International Classification of Diseases (ICD-10) protocol.

- *Patient examinations module*: This module keeps a record of all medical examinations, including obstetrical, gynecological, and clinical breast examinations and laboratory and radiological examinations. Through this module, the user can have access to the information related to any aforementioned examination, including diagnostic information, in a parameterization manner; the pharmaceutical treatment required; and/or any other specific medical instruction.

- *Obstetrical examination module*: This module manages all the obstetrical examination data. It contains all the necessary data related to the woman's pregnancy and labor. In particular, the module supports parameters during pregnancy and labor such as examinations of the placental, systolic, and diastolic arterial pressure; weight and temperature of the pregnant woman; start and end dates of the pregnancy; type of labor; number of fetuses; parameters of the fetus clinical examination; recording of problems related to the pregnancy and the labor; bone density measurements, etc. Furthermore, this module is connected to the *radiological test examinations module*, and it controls the image data related to any ultrasound examination.

- *Gynecological examination module*: This module manages all the gynecological examination data. It contains all the necessary information related to the clinical examination of gynecological organs such as cervix, uterus, fallopian tubes, ovaries, etc. Also, the module controls all clinical data related to any abdominal wall examination and vaginoscopy.

- *Gynecological operation module*: This module records the history of all gynecological operations per patient, based on the name of the patient and the date of her operation, along with all the corresponding clinical findings. The information controlled by this module includes the type and description of each operation, operational schemes (frontal anatomical, oblique anatomical, operational incisions, and external gynecological organs), pathological findings of fallopian tubes and ovaries, information related to possible implications, etc. The specific module also includes four different graphical "notebooks," which are developed by implementing computer graphics algorithms and correspond to the aforementioned four types of operational schemes. Through these graphical notebooks, the expert could easily draw and/or locate predefined operational findings such as inflammation, cyst, malignancy, fibromyoma, endometriosis, lymph node, and symphysis.

- *Laboratory examinations module*: This module records the results of various laboratory examinations, including blood tests, biochemical blood tests, urine tests, urine test culture, vaginal fluid examination, stool test, hormonical examinations, ions, cancer and hepatic markers, etc. All the laboratory examination parameters were coded using the ICD-10 protocol.

- *Pap smear module*: This module controls all the estimates related to the gynecological Pap smear, a test used for the early diagnosis of cancer of the uterus.

- *Clinical breast examination module*: This module holds all the information related to any clinical breast examination. It includes reasons for the specific examination, breast review (breast asymmetry, location, breast color, nipple status, etc.), breast palpation (location of a mass, characterization of the mass, etc.), pathological breast examination (excision and biopsy), and supplementary measurements (temperature, systolic and diastolic arterial pressure, etc.).

- *Radiological test examination module*: This module provides access to all data acquired from any medical imaging modality within the hospital. It implements the appropriate communication interfaces to the external systems such as PACS of the hospital or any other medical image-archiving system located at the radiology department, and it is connected wit the system's image processor for displaying, manipulating, and processing the data. Through this module, the system currently processes ultrasonic and mammographic images in DICOM format.

12.2.3
System Functionality

The development of the system, in terms of the interface, is focused toward the medical expert-user, it supports a number of users at the same time, and it is user-friendly and simple, requiring only knowledge of the Microsoft Windows environment. The main functionalities of the system are (1) management of the patient data and (2) processing and visualization of various gynecological data.

12.2.3.1
Management of Patient Data

The patient medical record is organized on three levels: (1) patients, (2) visits, and (3) various examinations–operations. The latter contains patient data related to various examinations (blood tests, radiological examination, clinical gynecological–obstetrical examination, and breast examination), other examinations (Pap smear, mammography, sperm examination), and surgical operations—deliveries.

Figure 12.3a shows a typical Web page of the patient data along with the main menu marked, whereas Fig. 12.3b shows the system's floating toolbar.

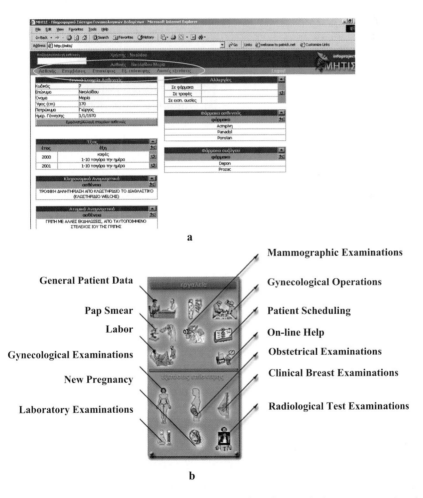

Fig. 12.3. a Typical Web page of recording patient data along with the main menu (*marked*).
b The system's floating toolbar

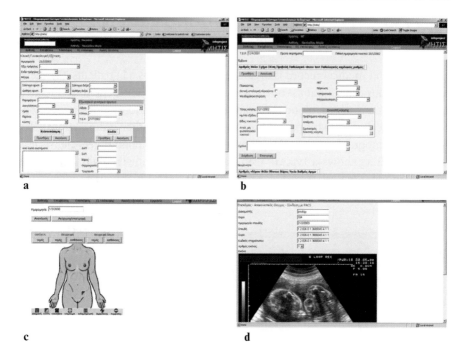

Fig. 12.4. Typical Web pages for **a** the gynecological examination, **b** the pregnancy/labor monitoring, **c** the frontal operational scheme applied along with the predefined findings/diseases using a graphical interface, and **d** the radiological test examination along with a typical ultrasonic image from the hospital's PACS in digital imaging and communications in medicine (DICOM) format

Also, Fig. 12.4 shows the typical Web pages for a gynecological examination (Fig. 12.4a), a pregnancy/labor monitoring examination (Fig. 12.4b), the frontal operational scheme applied along with the predefined findings/diseases using a graphical interface (Fig. 12.4c), and the radiological test examination along with a typical ultrasonic image from the hospital's PACS in DICOM format (Fig. 12.4d).

12.2.3.2
Image Processing and Viewing of Gynecological Data

This image processor provides all the capabilities for manipulating any gynecological images within the database (images in DICOM format), including image acquisition, display, image-saving capabilities in different image formats (Joint Photographic Experts Group, Tagged Image File Format, and Portable Network Graphics) and image processing. The image processor includes the following tools:

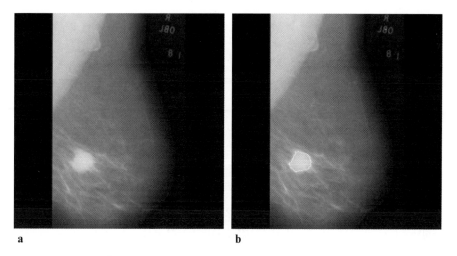

a   b

Fig. 12.5. Segmentation of pathological mammographic images: **a** the initial mammographic image and **b** the extracted contour of the region of interest (ROI) superimposed on the initial image using the proposed automatic morphology-based segmentation algorithm

- *Image enhancement tool*: It includes filters for histogram equalization, unsharp masking (Laplacian of a Gaussian), and contrast-limited adaptive histogram equalization [15].
- *Image segmentation tool*: This tool provides the specialist with the ability to isolate regions of interest (ROIs) in mammographic images, both manually and automatically. In the automatic approach, the segmentation of specific ROIs is performed by the development of an algorithm based on mathematical morphology [10]. The automatic algorithm was successfully applied to a number of pathological mammographic images where tumors like ROIs were automatically segmented, as shown in Fig. 12.5.

12.2.3.3
Classification of Mammographic Images

This module is a classification system of mammographic images, and a block diagram of the classification process is shown in Fig. 12.6. According to the diagram, each mammographic image is firstly processed by the image processor in order to extract specific ROIs, either automatically or manually. Then, the ROIs are further processed by the classification module.

The classification module comprises two submodules: the feature extraction module and the classifier. Features of the second-order statistics [6] were finally used, resulting in a final feature vector with dimensionality of 48. The classifier consists of a multilayer feed-forward artificial neural network (ANN) comprising

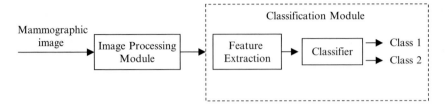

Fig. 12.6. The decision-support system for the classification of mammographic images

two layers of neurons: the input and the output layers [7]. The input layer consists of five neurons, whereas the output layer consists of one neuron, encoding the two classes of the ROIs: pathological and normal ROIs (0 represents pathological and 1 represents normal). The back-propagation algorithm with adaptive learning rate and momentum has been used in order to train the ANN [13]. During the experimental phase, 313 mammographic images (205 normal and 108 pathological) were used for the evaluation of the classification module. These images were selected from the MiniMammography database of the Mammographic Image Analysis Society, containing 320 digitized films, each of 1,024 × 1,024 pixels and 256 gray levels (8 bits) [16]. The 313 mammographic images involved in the study were finally chosen after thorough inspection by an experienced radiologist. All mammographic data used in the study were in portal gray map format. During the experimental phase, the overall classification rate achieved by the implementation of the proposed classification module was 93%. A comprehensive evaluation of methods of extraction of different features using the proposed classifier can be found in [10].

12.2.3.4
Registration of Mammographic Images

Another image-processing capability offered by the system is the registration of two mammographic images: one is called the reference and the other image is to be registered (in DICOM format), in order to evaluate a therapeutic scheme and/or to compare two examinations of the same patient at different times. Two registration methods have been incorporated within the system: (1) the manual method and (2) the automatic method. The *manual registration method* involves the selection of pairs of corresponding points in both images by the expert and the definition of any possible movements (displacements, rotations, etc.) by the application of an affine transformation on these corresponding points. The *automatic registration method* is based on the automatic identification and the spatial coincidence of the breast boundaries of the two

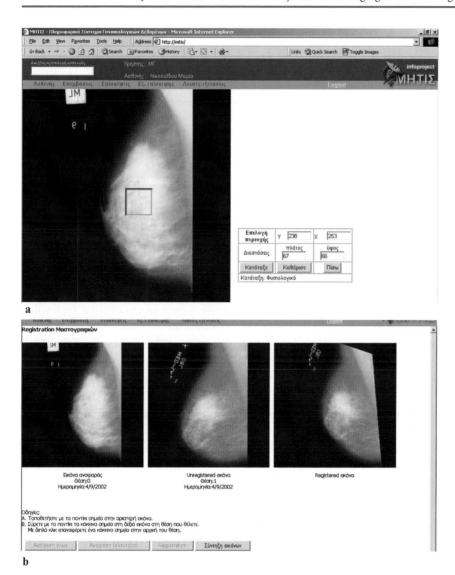

Fig. 12.7. Typical Web pages for **a** the classification of an isolated ROI within a mammographic image according to the decision-support system and **b** the registration of mammographic images

images using the affine transformation [14]. Both registration methods have been finally integrated into the system presented.

Figure 12.7 displays typical Web pages for the application of the image-processing algorithms developed. Figure 12.7a shows an isolated ROI within a mammographic image (locations and dimensions in pixels) along with the result of the classification process (normal–pathological) according to the decision-support system. The expert selected an ROI, which was then fed to the decision-support system, which classified the ROI as a normal. Figure 12.7b displays a representative result of the registration of mammographic images, as the registered image (right image), from the application of the automatic boundary-based registration algorithm between the reference image (left image) and the unregistered image (centered image). Furthermore, the system allows the fusion of the reference and the registered image for further evaluation of a therapeutic scheme or the progression of a disease.

12.2.4
System Security

The first step to establish secure communication was the use of password-based user authentication. Apart from this common username–password combination, the compatibility of the system with the Web permits the adoption of open and reliable user authentication and encryption technologies such as Secure Sockets Layer (SSL) to provide a secure communication channel between the server and the clients. The SSL is a standard protocol for secure Web transactions, and it operates on the basis of public and private keys.

Furthermore, Microsoft Windows 2000/IIS 5.0 was installed on the system to improve the security of Windows. All resources were placed on the Windows NT file system. The user verification procedure was based on both user information databases in the server and digital certificates from a mutually trusted third-party organization, such as VeriSign (http://www.verisign.com). Users are unable to access the programs unless they provide both correct login information and their digital certificates.

12.3
Clinical Application of the System

The system developed was installed in the "Alexandra" National Hospital, in Greece, for the pilot study in the last semester of 2004. Two departments within the hospital were able to successfully connect to the system, the gynecology and radiology departments sharing medical information. Since a PACS was not installed within the hospital, several alterations were made. The system was installed on a dedicated Web server in the gynecology department, and connections to both a digital mammography system and an ultrasound machine at the hospital's radiology department were made through a LAN. Since a number of private physicians cooperate with the hospital, five external gynecologists were successfully connected to the system using the Internet via fast ADSL connections. The system was also tested in terms of expert communication from the different departments as well as interaction of the information embedded in the system of the clinicians. Within a period of 2 months, a training program on the use and capabilities of the system was scheduled, involving two technicians and five physicians from the hospital and all five external physicians.

After a period of 5 months, when the system was under evaluation, more than 100 patients were recorded, and their examinations were successfully followed by the system, including various medical data. Also, the classification module was further tested for the classification of 40 mammographic images; 20 of those were characterized as normal and the rest as pathological, according to the specific clinical examinations. The classification module was able to correctly distinguish 18 out of the 20 (classification rate 90.0%) as normal and 16 out of the 20 as pathological (classification rate 80.0%). Thus, during the clinical implementation of the system, an 85.5% classification rate was achieved through the classification module for both categories.

12.4
Discussion

Since the system's pilot study, and for the last 2 years, the National Public Health System in Greece has undergone major changes. In particular, public hospitals and distant health centers all over Greece have been grouped into seven administrative sanitary regions, and efforts have been made toward the installation of unified hospital information systems (HIS), one at each region, connecting major hospitals via a wide-area network and rural health centers using Web technologies, to support the new planning. HIS, at present under development, are aiming to offer various services to the citizens using the Internet: examination scheduling, recording of daily examinations, home care support, billing capabilities, pharmaceutical warehouse management, support of bids within the hospitals, a laboratory information subsystem, a biomedical engineering subsystem for managing personnel and equipment, and an upper-level hospital management subsystem including control and reporting capabilities. In the Greek private health sector, similar systems have already been installed and operated in various hospitals, and they are currently being expanded to include external private physicians via Web technologies. The system presented could easily be incorporated within these HIS, sharing specific patient information, including various examinations, and providing services for the communication, management, and processing of images from radiology departments that are not supported by the HIS under development. On the other hand, the system presented could enhance communication of the public sector with private hospitals or individuals—experts for the delivery of better health services.

Two crucial factors for the successful integration of these HIS and any teleradiology system, such as the one presented, are the recruiting of appropriate personnel for operating and maintaining these systems and the education and training of personnel, both technical and medical. In our experience during the pilot study, these requirements will be difficult to meet in the public health sector unless specific actions such as reduction of the personnel's daily work load, improvement of the working environment, and economical motivation are taken. In contrast, in the private health sector, there is better provision of education and training opportunities, since efforts are taken to integrate general telemedicine and teleradiology applications in the daily clinical practice.

Nevertheless, academic training in teleradiology incorporates graduate or postgraduate courses in medical physics or biomedical engineering, which include short courses on telemedicine or health information systems with an emphasis on teleradiology, among other generic issues. Such courses are offered by several departments (e.g., the Department of Hygiene and Epidemiology of the Medical School at the University of Athens, the Department of Informatics of the University of Central Greece, etc.) as well as interdepartmental courses, such as the master of science in life science informatics with specialty in medical informatics, organized by the Medical School and the Biology Department of the University of Patras and other universities, and the graduate course in biomedical technology, organized by the Medical School of the University of Patras and the Department of Electrical and Computer Engineering of the National Technical University of Athens, in conjunction with other Greek universities.

Any possible uncovered needs in the education of teleradiology are usually tackled by vocational training of the professional involved. Vocational training in teleradiology is offered to all members of staff involved, by most product vendor companies or their regional representatives. The type of training varies from advanced extensive courses, which are dedicated courses that take place off site in formal classrooms, to on-the-job training, combined with final system installation, prior to acceptance testing. Usually, training is differentiated among system administrators, medical professionals, and members of the administration. It has to be emphasized, however, that software modules that support teleradiology have only penetrated public and private hospitals in Greece to a degree of no more than 3%.

In the near future, efforts will made to install the system presented in gynecology/obstetrics departments of hospitals and to connect it with existing HIS and/or those under development. Finally, the system presented is now fully operatational and is offered by Infoproject, a Greek software-development company.

12.5
Conclusions

A Web-based teleradiology medical system, called MITIS, has been developed for the management and processing of obstetrical, gynecological, and radiological medical data. The system, through its modular structure, records all the necessary medical information in terms of patient data, examinations, and operations and provides the user-expert with advanced image-processing tools for the communication, manipulation, processing, and storage of ultrasonic and mammographic images using the DICOM protocol. It can be installed in a hospital, bringing together medical experts from different fields such as gynecologists and radiologists within the hospital as well as gynecological experts located outside the hospital through the Internet.

Summary

- A comprehensive review of existing Web-based teleradiology systems was given in Sect. 12.1.
- Various technological scenarios along with criteria and scoring available during the development period of the system presented were analytically described verify the system's architecture used.
- An analytical description of a Web-based teleradiology system for managing and processing gynecological–obstetrical–radiological data was then presented. The description concerns the general system description, system architecture, and system functionalities. Typical Web pages showing the usage of the system were also included.
- A more comprehensive description of the system's functionality in terms of image processing of gynecological data and security issues was also presented.
- The results from the pilot application of the system were also included along with a discussion on issues related to the application of teleradiology systems in Greece and education and training opportunities at various centers in Greece.

References

1. Adelhard K (2001) Quality assurance of medical information in the Internet—challenges for a seal of approval in gynecology. Zentralbl Gynakol 123:458–45910
2. Bellazi R, Montani S, Riva A, Stefanelli M (2001) Web-based telemedicine systems for home care: technical issues and experiences. Comput Methods Progr Biomed 64:175–1871

3. Creighton C (1999) A literature review on communications between picture archiving and communication systems and radiology information systems and/or hospital information systems. J Digit Imaging 12:138–1437

4. Feingold M, Kewalramani R, Kaufmann GE (1997) Internet and obstetrics and gynecology. Acta Obstet Gynecol Scand 76:718–7248

5. Handles H, Busch C, Encarnacao J et al (1997) KAMEDIN: a telemedicine system for computer supported cooperative work and remote image analysis in radiology. Comput Methods Progr Biomed 52:175–1835

6. Haralick RM, Shanmugan K, Dinstein I (1973) Textural features for image classification. IEEE Trans Syst Man Cybern 3:610–62113

7. Haykin S (1994) Neural networks. MacMillan, New York

8. Horiil SC, Prior FW, Bidgood WD, Parisot C, Claeys G (1994) DICOM: an introduction to the standard. Radiology at the PennState Geisinger Medical Center, PennState Geisinger Medical Center. http://www.xray.hmc.psghs.edu/dicom/dicom_intro/index.html6

9. Laird SP, Wong JSK, Schaller WJ, Erickson BJ, de Groen PC (2003) Design and implementation of an Internet-based medical image viewing system. J Syst Soft 66:167–1812

10. Matsopoulos GK, Kouloulias V, Asvestas P, Mouravliansky N, Delibasis K, Demetriades D (2004) MITIS: a WWW-based medical system for managing and processing gynecological-obstetrical-radiological data. Comput Methods Progr Biomed 76:53–7112

11. McKeown MJ (1997) Use of the Internet for obstetricians and gynecologists. Am J Obstet Gynecol 176:271–2749

12. Olsen DR, Bruland OS, Davis BJ (2000) Telemedicine in radiotherapy treatment planning: requirements and applications. Radiother Oncol 54:255–2594

13. Press WH, Teukolsky SA, Vetterling WT, Flannery BP (1992) Numerical recipes in C: the art of scientific computing. Cambridge University Press, Cambridge

14. Richard FJP, Cohen LD (2003) A new image registration technique with free boundary constraints: application to mammography. Comput Vis Image Underst 89:166–19617

15. Stark AJ (2000) Adaptive image contrast enhancement using generalizations of histogram equalization. IEEE Trans Image Process 9:889–89611

16. Mammographic Image Analysis Society (2004) The MiniMammography database. http://www.wiau.man.ac.uk/services/MIAS16

17. Zeng H, Fei DY, Fu CT, Kraft KA (2003) Internet (WWW) based system of ultrasonic image processing tools for remote image analysis. Comput Methods Progr Biomed 71:235–2413

13

Robotized Tele-echography

Fabien Courreges, Pierre Vieyres, and Gerard Poisson

Abstract Intensive multidisciplinary research work has been carried out by several research teams, to improve every part of the tele-echography system. More recently, the efficiency of the diagnosis has also been proved, emphasizing the interest in the concept. Various conception approaches have been explored, for instance, to the robot design, according to the targeted usage. The design of a universal usage system is, however, very challenging owing to the constraints specification described in this chapter. Nevertheless, to date, the lightweight body-mounted robot design approach tends to satisfy the general use requirements. Improvement of the robot control has also permitted this kind of approach. Improvements to the other part of the teleoperation equipment have allowed the setting up in France of a medical center network equipped with on-duty tele-echography systems for real-time routine examination.

13.1
Introduction

One of telemedicine's major applications is providing skilled medical care to patients who are in some way isolated from the specialized care they need. This is especially the case for patients living in isolated areas with reduced or substandard medical facilities. Access to these services is only achieved through the use of dedicated applications, which allow remote expert consultations, providing faster responses in emergency or crisis situations. As ultrasound imaging is becoming more and more a part of emergency medical or surgical decision making, there is a greater need for this technique to be accessible in the majority of the isolated areas lacking ultrasound specialists. However, this specialized health-care method is a skilled and "expert-dependent" technique. Hence, in the last decade, several robotized telemedicine concepts and scenarios have been investigated [16, 17, 20]. Remote robotized echography, developed by the mobile tele-echography using an ultra-light robot (OTELO) European project consortium, is one possible solution that could satisfy this type of health-care need to benefit isolated populations. The principle is to provide a medical expert, located at a medical center, with the ability to remotely control in real time, kilometers or even hundreds of kilometers away, a robotic device handling an ultrasound probe on a distant patient, while at the same time ultrasound images are fed back to the expert. Ultrasound echography is a noninvasive and low-energy method, which is very well adapted for teleoperation without a patient safety issue.

To guarantee a reliable tele-examination and, therefore, diagnosis, it is important for the medical expert to forget about the distance between him/her and the patient. As a consequence, the remote-control accuracy of the robot, the replication of the expert gestures by the robot, and the quality and flow of the ultrasound images received are correlated elements. These are needed by the expert in the feedback-control loop of the overall robotized tele-echography chain and are necessary for the feasibility of the diagnosis.

The robot's mechanical design is based on the specifications provided by the medical end-users' specialty (e.g., abdominal, cardiac, or fetal), and the limitations of the actuators that contribute to the robot's weight, size, and dynamic performances. To the best of our knowledge, two mechanical approaches have been considered for these medical robots. One, as proposed in the MIDSTEP project, uses an existing industrial robot to hold the distant ultrasound probe [10]. The other uses dedicated lightweight robots based on either parallel or hybrid structure [6, 16, 20, 21]. Lightweight portable serial structures are the most promising to be rapidly available on the medical products market.

To date, while some advanced issues, such as haptic control, are still in a laboratory prototype state, several other critical issues have been resolved, allowing some systems to be already on duty with efficacy. The purpose of this chapter is to present in Sect. 13.2 the main parts of a tele-echography system. In Sect. 13.3, we discuss the requirements that should be satisfied by a tele-echography robotic system, emphasizing the capabilities offered by the latest scientific and technological innovations. Section 13.4 provides the results of the medical experimentation made with the OTELO robot.

13.2
Tele-echography Plant General Structure

A tele-echography plant is, above all, a teleoperation scheme; that is why it is made up of three main parts, as shown in Fig. 13.1, which corresponds to the OTELO project structure.

Let us describe these three parts:

1. *Master station or expert station*: This is the fixed control station located in an expert center where the ultrasound expert sends robot controls and is fed back with ultrasound images of the patient.

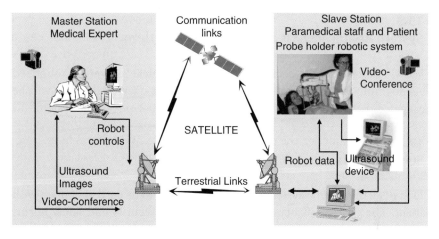

Fig. 13.1. Mobile tele-echography using an ultra-light robot (OTELO) tele-echography system

2. *Slave station or patient station*: This station may be mobile for an emergency or located in small clinics lacking ultrasound experts. It is made up of the robot with its control unit, an ultrasound imager, and paramedical staff to deploy the station, set up and supervise the remotely controlled examination, and assist the medical expert.
3. *Communication link*: This should ideally be versatile (terrestrial or by satellite, wired or wireless like the universal mobile telecommunications system).

As it is a multimodal application, one can identify four kinds of data to be transmitted:

1. *Synchronization flags*: These data are small bidirectional byte packets that are asynchronously transmitted. As the name says, these flags are used to synchronize the sequences of actions of the applications on both expert and patient sides. For instance, these flags are necessary for the initialization phase.
2. *Robot control data*: These data are also bidirectional for feedforward and feedback control of the robot.
3. *Videoconference data*: For a friendly usage and to allow the specialist to communicate with his/her patient assistant staff, a videoconferencing channel is necessary. These data are throughput-demanding but are not critical; consequently, a low quality of images and sound, provided by standard videoconferencing protocols, can be tolerated. Hence, the throughput required remains reasonable: 128 kbit/s is sufficient, as was shown in [14].
4. *Ultrasound images*: Theses are fed back to the expert from the robot site.

13.3
System Requirements and Technical Solutions

We will describe in this section the needs for an ideal "universal" robotized tele-echography system. That is to say that the stronger constraints will be investigated. Let us first analyze the needs on the robot side of the system.

13.3.1
Robot Design

First of all the robotic system must be safe, as it is to be used in contact with a patient. The system must conform to the medical security and safety norms (maternity, emergency, etc.):

- *Standard EN 60601-1, norm IEC 601, for the safety of use*: As the probe holder robot is dedicated to be in contact with persons (patient and medical assistant), it must be conceived to be easily and quickly held off the patient in the case of malfunction.
- *Electromagnetic interference among electronic devices must be avoided*: The electromagnetic compatibility in medicalized areas must satisfy the European norm EN 60601-1-2.

To satisfy the contact safety requirement, the French national research project TER (Robotized Tele-Echography) [7] led to the conception of an original robot intrinsically safe as its actuators were pneumatic braided; compliant artificial muscles were also named "rubbertuator" or "McKibben muscles."

The robotic equipment needs to be transportable to allow emergency intervention at isolated or hard-to-access areas. It should also be easily and rapidly set up in the case of emergency intervention.

The robot must be conceived to be able to mimic the expert's moves during an echography examination. To this end, the medical gestures of an ultrasound specialist have been monitored, in order to analyze the positions, trajectories, velocities (Fig. 13.2), and forces applied for various ultrasound investigations: cardiac, abdominal, and renal [2, 11].

The positioning of the patient must also be taken into account. Figure 13.3 shows the required probe positioning and the positions that the patient has to be set in for cardiac and abdominal examinations. Hence, the robot actuators subjected to gravity must be powerful enough to make the ultrasound probe track precisely the trajectories of the expert for any position of the patient.

During these specification studies, the following relevant points were reported:

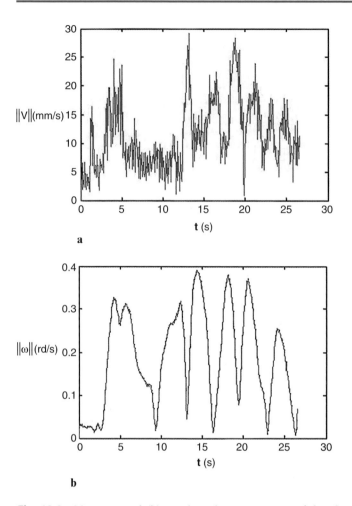

Fig. 13.2. (a) Linear and (b) angular velocity variations of the ultrasound probe during abdominal examination (liver)

- Continuous contact must be kept between the probe and the skin, even when the probe is applied on the ribs and irregular abdominal skin. This is an essential requirement to allow the penetration of the ultrasound and provide quality images.
- The contact force varies from 5 to 20 N.
- Once the probe has been positioned on the area of interest, rotations, inclinations, and small translations are performed around the chosen contact point with the skin (Fig. 13.4). From the design point of view, the robot has to perform rotations of the ultrasound probe around the contact point located

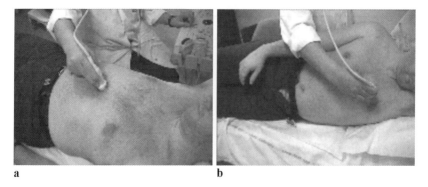

a   b

Fig. 13.3. Patient and ultrasound probe positioning during abdominal (**a**) and cardiac (**b**) examination

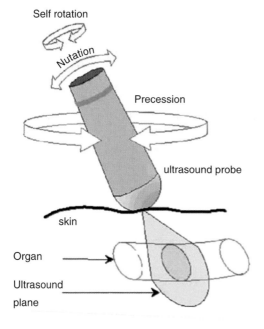

Fig. 13.4. Rotation moves of the ultrasound probe applied during an examination

outside the robotic structure. That is why this point is also called the "remote center of motion" (RCM).

- The probe axis is moved inside a conical space, and the axis of this cone is normal to the patient's skin (the angle between the probe axis and the normal direction to the skin is called nutation). The apex of this cone is the RCM. The probe is most often held close to the normal direction of the skin, except for some particular organs (bladder) or in the case of perinatal examina-

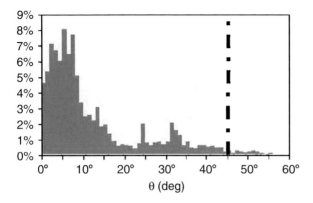

Fig. 13.5. Histogram of the ultrasound probe nutation values θ during a classic abdominal examination. The ordinates indicate the duration of the occurrence of the nutation. These durations are expressed as a percentage of the overall examination time

tions where the probe can be tilted up to a nutation of 60°. However, a vertex aperture of 45° can be considered as sufficient for most cases, according to the frequency of the nutation values shown in Fig. 13.5.

- An ultrasound probe generates an ultrasound plane (Fig. 13.4), and the medical expert has to rotate the probe properly around its own axis to observe the desired slice. As a consequence and according to the analysis of the movements, the robot should be able to apply every possible rotation to the probe inside the cone described above. To represent the attitude of the probe, let us consider the 3-1-3 Euler's angle system [15], composed of three angles: precession ψ, nutation θ, and self-rotation ϕ (Fig. 13.4). The previous requirement enables us to state that a complete coverage of 360° is necessary for the precession and self-rotation.

- The probe-holding system should be able to accept different kinds of ultrasound probe as different sizes of probe exist, adapted to the investigation of different organs.

All these previous requirements impose heavy constraints on the robot design. To date, few projects have been able to fully satisfy each constraint. However, the most promising approach is based on the conception of a mobile lightweight robotic device as in the OTELO project. Indeed, the concept proposed by this project consists of a small lightweight robot with a minimum number of actuators, which can be manually handled by a paramedic assistant on the patient's body. The assistant enables a gross placement of the robot on the patient, while the fine movements are remotely controlled by the medical expert.

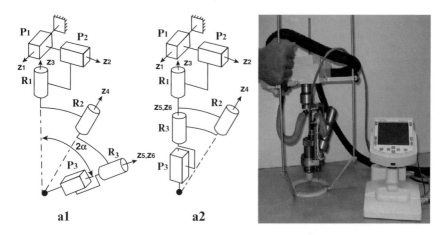

Fig. 13.6. OTELO robot kinematics

This kind of approach satisfies the constraints on contact safety and mobility for emergency intervention.

The robotic design of such a compact system is, however, delicate, since it must be able to track the expert's moves. The proposed robot kinematic (Fig. 13.6) offers an RCM. The ultrasound probe is rotated around the RCM by three actuated pivot joints: R1, R2, and R3. A force of up to 20 N on the patient can be exerted by a prismatic stepper motor P3. Two other actuated prismatic joints, P1 and P2, give the x–y degrees of freedom to the probe.

This kinematic has been proposed to fulfill every previous requirement concerning degrees of freedom and workspace.

While this kinematic exhibits mechanical singularities (configurations a1 and a2 in Fig. 13.6), it has been shown that suitable control laws for the robot enable an efficient and safe real-time examination of a remote patient even over very large distances [9]. A live feasibility demonstration was even done between France and Cyprus by satellite communication link.

Let us now analyze the requirements regarding the communication link and data transmission of a tele-echography system.

13.3.2
Communication and Data Transmission

The most critical data in this kind of application are the robot control and the ultrasound images.

Depending on the kind of robotic control chosen, the required throughput may vary greatly. As in this section we are discussing the requirements for

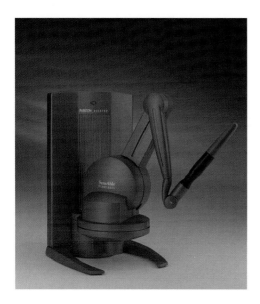

Fig. 13.7. PHANToM desktop haptic device

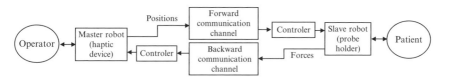

Fig. 13.8. Rudimentary force feedback control teleoperation scheme

worst-case conditions, we assume the communication link to be used is standard or even substandard. That is to say that the system should be able to work properly on a wide-area network like the Internet, with low guarantee of quality of service (QoS). In this case, a tradeoff has to be made on the choice of the robotic control: the higher the data rate, the more sophisticated and precise is the robot control, but less efficiently the network is capable of properly propagating the data (risks of loss, delay, or jitters). For example, let us assume that we want to have a force feedback control on the robot with a haptic input device provided to the expert. This kind of control enables the expert to feel the efforts as if he/she were applying the ultrasound probe on the patient. Indeed, the haptic device (such as the PHANToM interface from Sensable Technology, Fig. 13.7) handled by the expert is actuated so as to mimic the behavior of the patient's body.

Force sensors are to be implemented on the probe-holder robot to measure the efforts exerted on the patient. If we assume a classical force feedback control [4] such as in Fig. 13.8, the update rate of the robot control data shall be up to 1 kHz without loss or jitters, to render the teleoperation scheme "transparent" [18].

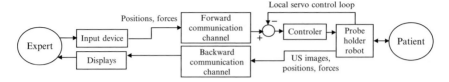

Fig. 13.9. OTELO teleoperation control scheme

"Transparency" means that the expert feels immersed. This can be hardly guaranteed on general networks. Moreover, as this kind of control is made up of a data feedback loop, it is very sensitive to delay and even more to jitters, which can cause the instability of the automated plant.

However, the benefits of this kind of control remain attractive and the adaptation of haptic control to low throughput and low QoS is being researched [12].

In the OTELO approach, the robot is open-loop-controlled over the communication link but locally closed-loop-controlled on the patient site (Fig. 13.9). This approach removes the control instability problem.

Moreover, it has been shown that the design of this robot enables the use of a geometric control [6]. That is to say, the robot can be precisely positioned by using a closed-form, fast-computable geometric model. This provides a major security advantage: when there is a communication cut, the robot only remains still at its last set-point position. This strong advantage allows the use of "lighter" network protocols without a data-recovering feature in the case of loss such as transmission control protocol, which has a heavy data frame overhead and may cause long unpredictable delays for recovery of lost data. Faster but more hazardous protocols can be used such as user datagram protocol or real-time transport protocol to enable the ultrasound specialist to perform a live remote echography. The low-bandwidth occupation of this kind of control has been shown on wireless networks [13].

The ultrasound images fed back to the expert are data of prime importance, as they constitute the expert diagnosis support and provide the expert with navigation information to drive the remote robot. Echography is a hand-to-eye coordination technique. When performing the telemedical act, the specialist mentally combines the position of the input device and the received patient ultrasound images to define both his/her current and next observation with respect to the organ investigated. Hence, in the robotized tele-echography chain, received ultrasound images provide the main information contributing to the feedback loop. They must be of the highest quality and delivered with a real-time flow, depending on to the communication link capability. To achieve such performance, the ultrasound images must be compressed before these are sent to the expert, so as to minimize the amount of data to be transmitted and the transmission time, while maintaining medical quality. Existing compression algorithms have been assessed for this kind of application [11], while some dedicated algorithms are under research [5]. One can identify two kinds of compression algorithms: algorithms with information loss and lossless algorithms. While lossless algorithms allow the original image to be recovered with all the information intact, the compression ratio remains low for real-time application. That is why algorithms of the first kind are preferably investigated by removing the useless information (noise) in the image.

13.3.3
Human–Machine Interfaces

The tele-echography scheme is dedicated to strong interaction and cooperation with the teleoperation staff. As a consequence, interfaces must be friendly, ergonomic, immersive, and quickly understandable.

We investigate two main interface spots:

1. *At the expert site*: The medical expert must be provided with an input device to drive the remote robot. He/she should also be able to communicate with his/her patient and to visualize the ultrasound images received. While these latter requirements can be fulfilled with existing videoconferencing systems and displays, providing an input device for robot control is not trivial. Various approaches have been investigated: in the majority of the tele-echography projects, general-use interfaces have been employed. For instance, Abolmaesumi et al. [1] use a joystick and Guerraz [18] uses a commercial PHANToM haptic device. However, it has been shown that dedicated interface props are best suited for immersion [19]. An interface prop is an instrumented input device resembling the actual device to be handled when the operator directly performs his/her task. For an echography task, the device to be handled is the ultrasound probe. Hence, for tele-echography, the interface prop should look like an ultrasound probe. This is the approach of Poisson et al. [22], who proposed a patented input device dedicated to tele-echography, called a "fictive probe." It is a hands-free input device, allowing the medical expert to perform natural medical gestures as in conventional conditions (Fig. 13.10a). This device is fitted with a force sensor and a 6D localization magnetic sensor giving the attitude and position of the fictive probe in real time. These sensors provide the set points for the robot control. Moreover, the fictive probe is a passive pseudohaptic device, as a spring mounted inside makes the operator feel as though he/she is applying effort on a patient's body. The last patented version of the fictive probe makes it become an active haptic

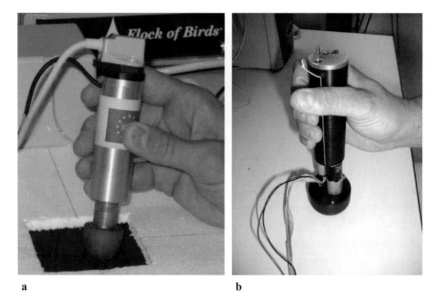

a   b

Fig. 13.10. Patented fictive probes: **a** passive and **b** active

device, since an actuator is integrated inside. The actuator can therefore be controlled to render to the expert the effort sensed by the robot on the patient (Fig. 13.10b).

2. *At the patient site*: There is a mechanical interaction between the robot and the patient. For body-mounted robots, such as the OTELO or TER robots, the mounting interface must be carefully designed. Indeed, the robot support on the patient must not be painful even after a long examination and should adapt to any part of the body to be examined. Experiments have shown that a ring-shaped support (Fig. 13.6) with a sufficiently large contact surface (dimensioned according to the robot weight) guarantees a painless examination even for pregnant women.

13.4
Clinical Results

The following reported experiments are published results from the OTELO project [8].

The tele-echography system was tested at two hospitals with different medical experts. The first was the hospital Trousseau of Tours in France. Tests were performed by an expert situated in a different room from the patient.

Two integrated services digital network (ISDN) lines connected the two sites. One line (128 kbit/s) was allocated for video transmission (switching between the video from a room camera and the video from the ultrasound scanner) and one channel in the other line (64 kbit/s) was allocated for robotic data. Tele-ultrasound examinations were performed on 20 patients to obtain longitudinal and transverse views of the heart and intra-abdominal organs.

The second hospital was the Corporacio Sanitaria Clinic in Barcelona (Spain). Tele-ultrasound examinations were performed by an expert situated approximately 3 km from the patient station located in the hospital clinic.

Examinations were performed on 32 individuals (16 control subjects and 16 patients). Twenty-two examinations were done using three ISDN connections at a maximum bandwidth of 384 kbit/s. Ten examinations were done with a satellite (Eultelsat) connection. The satellite link provided an average bandwidth of approximately 284 kbit/s. Three ultrasound scanners were used: 14 individuals with a Tringa, 12 individuals with a Toshiba Just-Vision, and six individuals with a Toshiba SAL 140D. A complete abdominal examination was performed.

At both test sites, the views obtained by the remote robotic device were compared with those obtained from a standard ultrasound examination performed directly on the patient with a more modern ultrasound device. The results are summarized in Table 13.1 as a comparison rate of the tele-examination to the standard examination.

Table 13.1. Performance results of the tele-echography scheme with respect to a standard examination performed as a reference

	Mean examination duration (min)	Posttraumatic disorders (aorta, kidneys, liver, spleen, and bladder) (%)	Four-chamber heart views (%)	Digestive symptoms (liver, gall bladder, pancreas, and kidney) (%)	Urinary/ pelvis symptoms (bladder, kidney, prostate, uterus, and ovaries) (%)	Lesions (%)
Trousseau Hospital	24	80	90	100	100	×
Corporacio Sanitaria Clinic	21	85	×	>64	100	66

A *cross* indicates the study was not carried out.

The difficulty in identifying lesions was due to low resolution (eight individuals), suboptimum scanning related to the new technical application (three individuals), inadequate image transmission (seven individuals), or poor patient health (one individual).

Except for some difficulties due to the particular conditions described above, the diagnosis obtained with the remote scanning system agreed in approximately 80% of the cases with the diagnosis made by conventional scanning. These results greatly justify the usage of a robot compared with other tele-ultrasound techniques, such as those consisting of the acquisition of ultrasound images performed directly on a patient by an expert and transmitted, after completion of the examination, through an ISDN connection to a remote expert assessing the quality of the ultrasound images received. The results using this latter technique [3] indicated a diagnostic acceptability of only 20%.

Hence, the previous results demonstrate the feasibility and efficiency of robotized tele-echography.

13.5
Conclusions and Perspectives

Since 1998, the technical feasibility of robotized tele-echography has been demonstrated. From that date, intensive multidisciplinary research work has been carried out by several research teams, to improve every part of the tele-echography system. More recently, the efficiency of the diagnosis has also been proved, emphasizing the interest in the concept. Various conception approaches have been explored, for instance, to the robot design, according to the targeted usage. The design of a universal usage system is, however, very challenging owing to the constraints specification described in this chapter. Nevertheless, to date, the lightweight body-mounted robot design approach tends to satisfy the general use requirements. Improvement of the robot control has also permitted this kind of approach. Improvements to the other part of the teleoperation equipment have allowed the setting up in France of a medical center network equipped with on-duty tele-echography systems for real-time routine examination.

Improvements to come will be to the robot design by using lighter and more resistant materials for size reduction. The robot design can also benefit from a deeper analysis of the medical experts' moves during standard examinations. Consequential work is in progress for transparent haptic teleoperation. This work will result in advances in robot control under time-varying delays and in force feedback interfaces that will benefit tele-echography.

Summary

The points discussed in this chapter are as follows:

- Robotized tele-echography concept and architecture
- Robotized tele-echography applications and perspectives
- Requirements for robotized tele-echography
- OTELO project innovations
- Clinical validation with the OTELO system

References

1. Abolmaesumi P, Sirouspour MR, Salcudean SE, Zhu WH (2001) Adaptive image servo controller for robot-assisted diagnostic ultrasound. Paper presented at the IEEE/ASME international conference on advanced intelligent mechatronics (AIM), Como
2. Al Bassit L (2005) Structures mécaniques à modules sphériques optimisées pour un robot médical de télé-échographie mobile. PhD thesis, University of Orléans
3. Brebner JA, Ruddick-Bracken H, Brebner EM et al (2000) The diagnostic acceptability of low-bandwidth transmission for tele-ultrasound. J Telemed Telecare 6:335–338
4. Buss M, Schmidt G (1998) Control problems in multi-modal telepresence systems. Institute of Automatic Control Engineering, Technische Universität München, Munich, pp 66–101
5. Capri A (2007) Caractérisation des objets dans une image en vue d'une aide à l'interprétation et d'une compression adaptée au contenu : application aux images échographiques. PhD thesis, University of Orléans
6. Courrèges F (2003) Contributions à la conception et commande de robots de télé-échographie. PhD thesis, University of Orléans
7. Courreges F, Poisson G, Vieyres P, Vilchis-Gonzales A, Troccaz J, Tondu B (2002) Low level control of antagonist artificial pneumatic muscles for a tele-operated ultrasound robot. Paper presented at ISMCR'02—12th international symposium on measurement and control in robotics, Bourges
8. Courreges F, Vieyres P, Istepanian RSH, Arbeille P, Bru C (2004) Clinical trials and evaluation of a mobile tele-echography robotic system. JTT J Telemed Telecare 11(Suppl 1): 46–49
9. Courreges F, Vieyres P, Poisson G, Novales C (2005) Real-time singularity controller for a tele-operated medical ecography robot. Paper presented at IROS2005, IEEE/RSJ international conference on intelligent robots and systems, Edmonton
10. De Cunha D, Gravez P (1998) The MIDSTEP system for ultrasound guided remote tele-surgery. In: 20th annual intelligent of the IEEE/EMBC Engineering in Medicine and Biology Society, vol 20, no 3. Hong Kong, pp 1266–1269
11. Delgorge C, Courreges F, Al Bassit L et al (2005) A tele-operated mobile ultrasound scanner using a light weight robot. IEEE Trans Innov Technol Biomed. 9(1):50–58
12. Fonte A, Courreges F, Mourioux G, Slama T, Vieyres P, Poisson G (2005) Stability and transparency for robotised tele-echography under time-delay : a preliminary study. Paper presented at REM2005, 6th international workshop on research and education in mechatronics, Annecy, France

13. Garawi SA, Courreges F, Istepanian RSH, Gosset P, Zisimopoulos H (2004) Performance analysis of a compact robotic tele-echography e-health system over terrestrial and mobile communication links. Paper presented at IEE 3G 2004, 5th international conference on 3G mobile communication technologies, London

14. Gilabert R, Vannoni M, Courreges F et al (2004) Clinical validation of a tele-operated mobile ultrasound scanner using a light weight robot (OTELO project). Poster presented at ECR 2004, European Congress of Radiology, Vienna

15. Goldstein H (1980) Classical mechanics, 2nd edn. Addison-Wesley, Reading

16. Gonzales AV, Cinquin P, Troccaz J et al (2001) A system for robotic tele-echography. In: Proceedings of medical image computing and computer-assisted intervention, MICCAI 200114-17. Lecture notes in comput science, vol 2208. Springer, Heidelberg, pp 326–334

17. Gourdon A, Vieyres P, Poignet Ph, Szpieg M, Arbeille Ph. (1999) A tele-scanning robotic system using satellite communication. IEEE/EMBEC 99, European Medical and Biological Engineering Conference, Vienna, Austria

18. Guerraz A (2002) Etude du télégeste médical non invasif utilisant un transducteur gestuel à retour d'efforts. PhD thesis, Université Joseph-Fourier, Grenoble I

19. Hinckley K, Pausch R, Goble JC, Kassell NF (1994) Passive real-world interface props for neurosurgical visualization. In: Proceedings of CHI' 94, pp. 452–458

20. Masuda K, Kimura E, Tateishi N, Ishihara K (2001) Three dimensional motion mechanism of ultrasound probe and its application for tele-echography system. In: Proceedings of the 2001 IEEE/RSJ International conference on intelligent robots and systems. Piscataway, NJ: IEEE, pp 1112–1116

21. Najafi F (2004) Design and prototype of a robotic system for remote palpation and ultrasound imaging. MSc thesis, University of Manitoba, Winnipeg

22. Poisson G, Vieyres P, Courreges F, Smith-Guerin N, Novales C (2003) Ultrasound probe simulator. European Patent EP1333412

14

US Army Teleradiology: Using Modern X-ray Technology To Treat Our Soldiers

David M. Lam, Kenneth Meade, Ronald Poropatich, Ricanthony Ashley, and Edward C. Callaway

Abstract This chapter briefly discusses the early use of military radiology and then concentrates on the developments that have taken place since the Vietnam War. Lighter, more robust field X-ray units, using digital computed radiography, have replaced film and wet processing, allowing rapid transmission of these digital images to supporting tertiary-care medical facilities continents away for interpretation (teleradiology). Along with the development of the communication infrastructure needed to support this utilization, these changes have forever altered the concept of military combat radiology. These changes are now becoming institutionalized and will form the framework for future collaboration between the Veterans Health Administration and the military medical services.

14.1
Introduction

Almost immediately after the seminal article in 1896 by Roentgen [21] on the potential medical use of X-rays, military physicians began to make use of this novel modality.

In 1896, an Italian physician, LTC Alvaro, used X-rays to locate bullets in casualties of the war in Ethiopia. However, his work was done far from the front, in Naples [3].

X-rays were used on both sides during the Greco–Turkish war of 1897 and X-ray units were located in temporary military hospitals still well separated from the front [1, 2, 12]. The X-ray apparatus of these early days was heavy and fragile and was limited by the lack of reliable power supplies (Fig. 14.1). Ships' generators and bicycles were only two of the methods used to recharge the batteries. Images were usually produced on glass negatives, using wet chemistry.

The first actual uses of X-rays near a fighting front were reported by Beevor [5] and Battersby [4], who reported separately on their utilization on the front lines in 1898. Operational requirements precluded moving the wounded from the front, so neither Beevor nor Battersby had the luxury of establishing himself in safe havens.

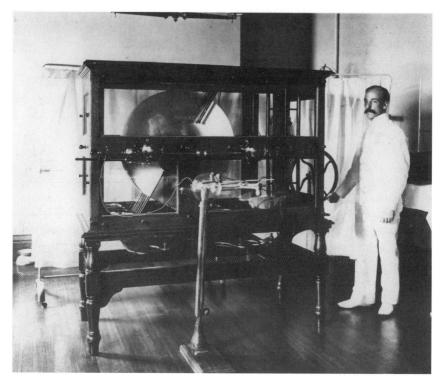

Fig. 14.1. Otis Clapp X-ray machine circa 1896. (Courtesy of the National Museum of Health and Medicine, Armed Forces Institute of Pathology, Washington, AMM 3712)

As a result of these experiences, the US military rapidly deployed X-ray units during the Spanish–American War of 1898, although only to fixed-base hospitals and to three deployed hospital ships (Fig. 14.2). There was a consensus that deploying X-ray units too close to the front would only encourage physicians to carry out surgery under unfavorable conditions of limited asepsis. As a result of this operational experience, Captain William Borden carried out a study of the use of X-rays, examining various types of X-ray apparatus, and recommended the coil apparatus over the static types for military use because the former were unaffected by the environment, were more portable, were cheaper to maintain, and suffered less breakage in use [6].

Radiology advanced little in the US military until World War I, being restricted to use in hospital ships and fixed-base hospitals, but the war in Europe saw the X-ray machine deployed to far-forward surgical hospitals, aided by technological advances, which made the machines more usable in the field (Fig. 14.3). These advances included improved power sources, the Coolidge hot filament X-ray tube, and X-ray film that replaced the previously used fragile and heavy glass plates. Truck-mounted machines powered by gasoline generators became standard (Fig. 14.4) [11].

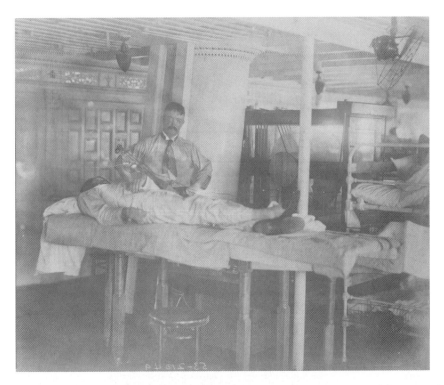

Fig. 14.2. X-rays on hospital ship relief, Spanish–American War. (Courtesy of the National Museum of Health and Medicine, Armed Forces Institute of Pathology, Washington, AMM 2186)

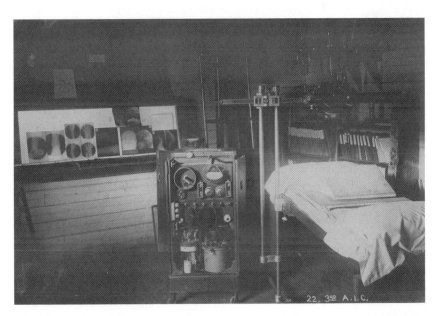

Fig. 14.3. World War I (WWI) X-ray installation at Issoudon, France. (Courtesy of the National Museum of Health and Medicine, Armed Forces Institute of Pathology, Washington, Reeve 11669)

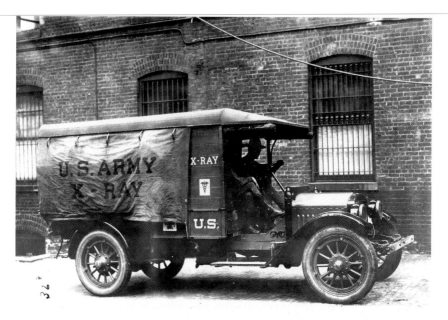

a

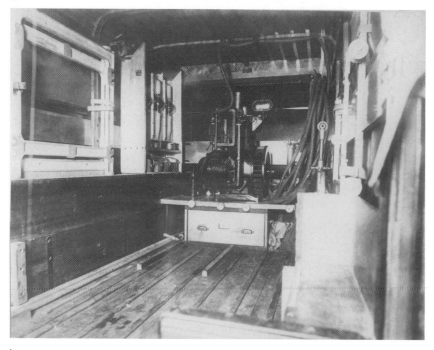

b

Fig. 14.4. US Army truck-mounted X-ray unit, WWI: **a** exterior and **b** interior. (Courtesy of the National Museum of Health and Medicine, Armed Forces Institute of Pathology, Washington, Reeve 13315 and 13316)

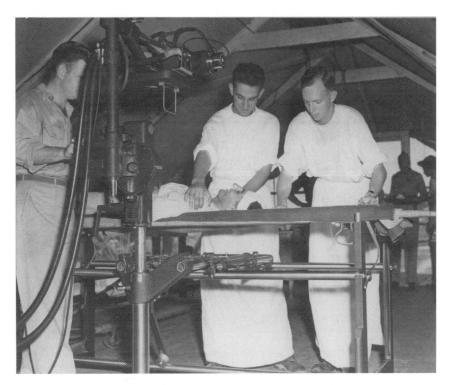

Fig. 14.5. X-rays in the field setting, 1942. (Courtesy of the National Museum of Health and Medicine, Armed Forces Institute of Pathology, Washington, SC 139639)

This technological development continued during the interwar period, resulting in lighter-weight equipment that was provided to all field hospitals (Fig. 14.5). However, there was no significant technological development in field X-ray machines (except for increased exposure protection) until the Vietnam War, during which high-power machines were fielded to brigades and hospitals. The deployable medical system of this later period included containerized radiological suites, including some portable fluoroscopic equipment, circa 1965–1970 (Fig. 14.6). Operation Desert Storm in 2001 saw the development of field-usable CAT scanners, which were provided to several of the deployed combat support hospitals (CSHs).

14.2
Overview of Current Military Radiology

Deployable digital radiography is now increasingly in use with many national armed forces, perhaps mostly by those of the USA. With over nine million beneficiaries located in both fixed and deployed settings around

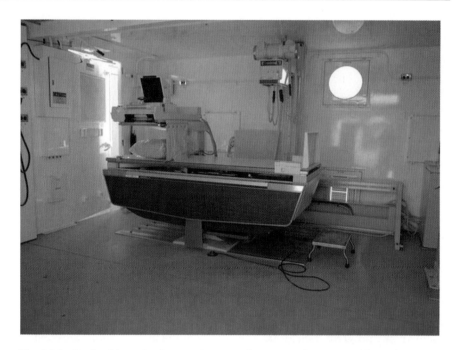

Fig. 14.6. Deployable medical system X-ray machine, 1986. (Courtesy of the Defense Visual Information Center, DM-SC-87-01658)

the world, both active duty and civilian—unlike any other country's scope/ needs or magnitude, the US military has been a strong proponent of digital radiography for more than 15 years. Building on lessons learned from the war in Vietnam and other deployed missions that followed, the US military embarked on a significant program for the improvement of military radiology. The goals were to improve reliability, decrease logistics support requirements, eliminate "wet processing" of films, and eventually centralize radiological interpretation and storage at sites remote from the battlefield, through the use of teleradiology. This effort has been led by the US Army PACS Program Management Office (APPMO) at the US Army Medical Research and Materiel Command (USAMRMC), with the Telemedicine and Advanced Technology Research Center (TATRC) and its predecessor organizations leading the way.

Since initial implementation, the technology used has gone through numerous changes, but it has kept up with the current state of the art. Today's systems include Web-based programs, leased landlines, and very small aperture terminal (VSAT) satellite terminal connectivity in remote deployed locations. Not all facilities have the same capabilities, but generally they are provided with Internet connectivity, digital still cameras, videoconferencing equipment, and digital radiology. All facilities are connected to the military's medical information management network, the Armed Forces Health Longitudinal Technology Application (AHLTA). Picture archiving and communication systems (PACS) are located at various points in the system to allow rapid transfer and archiving of images. Teleradiology has become the routine way of accomplishing radiology in the US military both in garrison and in deployed settings.

Little was accomplished in the military with regard to telemedicine (TMED)/ teleradiology during the years immediately following the Vietnam War. However, with increasing small-unit deployments around the world, it became obvious in the 1990s that not every mission could be supported with the entire panoply of medical support that had been developed for use in Vietnam.

In 1992, after an evaluation as to potential mechanisms for decreasing the size and complexity of the deployed medical force, it was decided that TMED would be one of the mainstays of future military medical deployments and that teleradiology, specifically, would be an integral part of this program. Accordingly, in July 1993, the Chief of Staff of the Army approved the establishment of the Army Telemedicine program. One of the earliest teleradiology programs deployed to US military forces in Europe was the Remote Clinical Communications System (RCCS) program, initiated by the Army Medical Department (AMEDD) Chief Information Officer's office in December 1992 and then implemented beginning in May1993 by the Medical Advanced Technologies Management Office (MATMO), the predecessor to the US TATRC at Fort Detrick, Maryland. The RCCS was intended to connect all peacetime garrison hospitals and clinics in Europe, as well as all deployed US Army forces in the European theater. This system provided communications through international maritime satellite (INMARSAT) systems and dedicated high-speed landlines, with the main station at Landstuhl Regional Medical Center (LRMC), Germany.[1] Radiology support during this program was achieved by transmission of digitized hard-copy film images. This system of teleradiology proved to be successful, although far from optimum. Speed of transmission and quality of transmitted images were less than desirable, and it was not well received by the clinicians in the outlying clinics [13]. (It must be noted that the RCCS was primarily used in 1993 and 1994 with a Kodak digital camera for teleconsultation, most of which did not include radiology images.)

---

[1] During the period covered by this chapter, the Landstuhl Army Regional Medical Center was renamed the Landstuhl Regional Medical Center (LRMC) to reflect its joint service nature rather than its previous incarnation as an Army-specific facility. Throughout this chapter it will be referred to as LRMC to preclude confusion.

The development of the imaging-standard digital imaging and communication in medicine (DICOM) facilitated radiological digital storage on PACS in the early 1980s. This created significant improvements in the ways in which images could be taken, stored, and transmitted for interpretation. The MATMO began to install the medical diagnostic imaging support (MDIS) system in 1994, which provided PACS and teleradiology at multiple medical treatment facilities (MTFs) throughout the USA and abroad. The goals of the MDIS project were to improve patient care, maximize limited resources, and realize cost savings—numerous lessons were learned in the areas of image quality, speed of image transmission, communication between sites, and the advantages of the MDIS two-way teleradiology configuration [16, 17, 19]. Those "lessons learned" led the Army to believe that teleradiology provided enough benefit that the RCCS and MDIS programs were expanded to include US medical elements located in Macedonia and Croatia in support of the United Nations Protection Force mission in the former Yugoslavia, as well as in Somalia [7].

14.3
Balkan Operations

After the formation of the TATRC in 1995, and with the increased activities of US forces in the Balkan region, the RCCS was extended as the project Prime Time to provide TMED support to US forces throughout the Former Yugoslav Republic of Macedonia, Bosnia-Herzegovina, and later Kosovo. When the US government deployed forces to Bosnia-Herzegovina as a part of the NATO Implementation Force in 1995, a full complement of military medical support facilities was established near Tusla, Bosnia. Smaller bases in the region then had their radiology services supported by the Prime Time project. The Prime Time program integrated these older technologies into the operating TMED system through the use of a "rapid prototyping" method, which enabled us to "push the envelope" as a technique for rapidly assessing both new technology and new operating concepts simultaneously as part of an overall fast-track concept exploration and validation process. This approach was initiated in advanced development situations in which more traditional research and development approaches could not keep pace with the tempo of rapidly evolving technology and doctrine such as high-bandwidth telecommunications and digital imaging. In 1995, the Imaging Science and Information Systems Center at Georgetown University contracted with the TATRC to develop an improved deployable teleradiology system (DTRS), which was desired to provide radiology support to areas that had radiology imaging capability but no direct access to a radiologist. Their efforts were focused on development of a digital imaging network (DIN) and PACS. In less than 3 months, the required system was designed, developed, and deployed by integrating 11 vendors' equipment and standard off-the-shelf components, integrated by use of the DICOM-3 standard. The deployable radiology system was installed at a CSH in Hungary, the Mobile Army Surgical Hospital (MASH) in Bosnia, and the LRMC in Germany in April 1996 [15, 18]. A major new aspect of this system was the use of filmless radiography in most locations—the first time such capability had been deployed to a military setting. Satellite, microwave, and high-speed landlines were used for communication between the three sites, and computed radiography (CR) and dry film printing replaced film development. On the basis of clinical experience, communications remained a combination of landline (leased E-1 lines) and satellites, with VSATs slowly replacing the expensive and low-bandwidth INMARSAT terminals previously used (Fig. 14.7) [9]. From 1995 to 1997, more than 20,000 digital diagnostic examinations (CR; computed tomography, CT; and ultrasound) were acquired, transferred, and archived using this system. The success of this teleradiology network prompted the US Army to consider and arrange for deployment of similar technologies in other parts of the world where troops are deployed. Since then this work has evolved into a global teleradiology network to support deployed US troops.

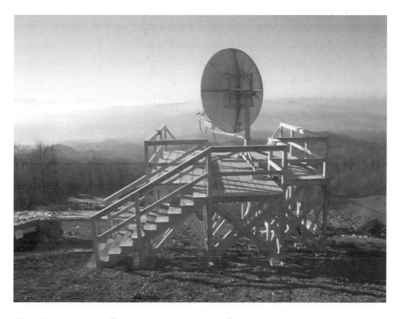

Fig. 14.7. Very small aperture terminal installation at Camp Morgan, Bosnia, 2001. (Photo courtesy of Kenneth Meade)

14.4
Kosovo and the ERMC DIN–PACS

Teleradiology in Kosovo cannot be discussed without mention of the US Army and the LRMC DIN-PACS. In 2002, the LRMC began using the satellite TMED network, which existed between Kosovo and Landstuhl, for reading clinical films that were generated by patient visits at both the locations. On October 21, 2002, the LRMC PACS was connected to Kosovo, and then to Bosnia on December 10, 2002. The teleradiology connection between the facilities enabled bidirectional transmission of DICOM images, facilitated by a commercial DICOM server (Medweb, San Francisco, CA, USA) at each of these sites. This capitalized on the fact that there was a clinical requirement to have a radiologist deployed in Kosovo. Although for considerations on quality of care this deployment was necessary, the radiological workload in Kosovo was quite minimal, and the skills of this radiologist could then be used to read films that were taken of patients in the garrison clinics in Germany. This activity now goes on routinely and is similar to what is being done in the civilian community [2]; but, at the time of its inception, it represented a unique step forward in the optimal usage of deployed military medical manpower. One anecdotal success story using the equipment came from a radiologist who had been working in the continental USA. The radiologist's deployment left the department short of physicians ; the radiologist was able to provide continued support to the department by reading the films that were generated during the night shift in the USA (which was daytime for the radiologist in Kosovo). This example highlights the need for a distributed medical network, the leveraging of scarce medical resources, and taking advantage of the "awake clock" for a military system that spans many time zones.

The Kosovo hospital operation has continued to the present date and is still manned by a radiologist who spends the majority of the working day reading films that have been generated by Army health facilities in Germany. The majority of these radiologists are military reserve physicianss who generally have somewhat limited experience with the Army PACS. They are rotated on a 3-month basis; prior to deploying to Kosovo, they stop by Landstuhl for a few days of training. Occasionally, it becomes necessary to provide staff assistance visits to their hospital to assist with problems. The system works well; much of this success can be attributed to the fact that since the Kosovo hospital's medical automation system is a node of Landstuhl's system, there are minimal difficulties with filling out the patient demographic DICOM header properly and the voice-generated dictations are smoothly integrated into the system. This contrasts with the operations in Iraq and Afghanistan described in the following sections, where the lack of this level of coordination leaves many films without adequate identifying data and/or difficulties with connecting the dictation and film in the PACS.

14.5
Afghanistan (Operation Enduring Freedom)

As a result of lessons learned in the Balkans, an effort was made to develop a standardized teleradiology system for deployment [10]. The DTRS, a commercial off-the-shelf product (Medweb, San Francisco, CA, USA), was investigated and purchased. The DTRS is a Web-based teleradiology product with unusually robust and secure communication capabilities. It also provides the capability for immediate local distribution of digital medical images throughout a fixed or mobile medical facility, provides historical archiving of images, and ensures secure transmission of images between medical facilities for interpretation and/or subspecialty consultation. The DTRS servers provide the physical hardware hub and information-processing center for all radiology systems and services within the deployed CSH. Residing on the CSH's local-area networks (LAN), medical diagnostic images and patient information will be stored locally and then securely transmitted to higher echelons of care as patients are transited from the theater hospital to sustaining base medical centers.

In December 2001, military operations of the US and coalition forces were established at Bagram, Afghanistan. Initial hospitalization support was provided by a Spanish medical unit, but in the summer of 2002 this was replaced by a US Army CSH. An assessment of regional TMED needs had been requested earlier by the Army Surgeon General, LTG James Peake; the results of this survey had suggested that teleradiology could enhance the medical care that was to be provided at this site. On the basis of LRMC's success in Bosnia and Kosovo, and in consultation with the APPMO, the TATRC, Fort Detrick deployed the DTRS to the 339th CSH in Afghanistan in October 2002 as part of Operation Enduring Freedom (OEF). In late October 2002, a small group was sent to Afghanistan by the TATRC and the Surgeon General's Office, which included a physician as officer in charge, a medical administrative officer, and several technical support individuals. Through the use of commercially purchased bandwidth, this team established a network connection between the deployed CSH hospital in Bagram, Afghanistan, and the LRMC in Germany, which was capable of transmitting complete DICOM images from the local PACS by use of the commercially available DICOM servers.

The initial operational concept was that this connection would make films available for consultation and would provide a means to forward images of patients scheduled for evacuation. It would also provide the ability to permanently archive images. The initial efforts were not as successful as desired. The supported radiologist and physicians had little interest in ordering second-opinion consultations, and the number of patients who were being evacuated at this time was small. Numerous technical difficulties relating to firewalls, network management, reliable satellite availability, and bandwidth resulted in an initial experience that was perceived as disappointing. In the absence of a strong desire from the deployed facility to maintain the service, the usage fell below expectation. It was not until later in the war when the deployed radiology services began to more seamlessly reproduce usual hospital practices that the project could be declared more successful.

Since the initial usage was less than that hoped for—during the first year of operation, teleradiology at this site did not gain strong support from the providers on the ground—it was sometimes perceived as unnecessary. Additionally, difficulties with the reliability of image transmission existed. Since Bagram teleradiology did not generate clinical usage metrics that could provide support for the expense of the equipment and bandwidth, it was difficult to justify the expense of the program.

The teleradiology system in Afghanistan has not achieved the same degree of success that has been noted in the Iraq theater (see Sect. 14.6), for several reasons. This operation has been multinational, and the numbers of US casualties in this theater are smaller, thus creating an environment in which it has been more difficult to perfect and validate work processes that facilitate automatic inclusion of the patient demographic information necessary for identifying DICOM images. In a recent week, about 1,300 images were forwarded from Afghanistan to the LRMC for archiving, and additional studies are forwarded routinely in coordination with evacuation for treatment of medical conditions. This is substantially less than the usage presently being recorded from Iraq. The relative numbers of images transmitted tend to vary depending on whose soldiers are combatants in Afghanistan; when the Canadians were involved, many were being sent to the LRMC for care, and this created a high demand—other nations routinely evacuate their casualties to non-US facilities in their home countries, thus reducing the need to transmit radiographs to the LRMC. The fact that a US Air Force facility is operating the hospital at the time of this writing has also been a factor. Our experience has been that Army facilities have been easier to integrate into the Army-operated LRMC system than are other services.

As a final remark on the struggles that have occurred with providing teleradiology to Bagram, it must be noted that our conclusion is that a successful system in this environment must be (1) medical standard of care, (2) undisputedly able to save lives, or (3) of demonstrated benefit from a cost–benefit viewpoint. During the early phases of operation, the teleradiology system met none of these three provisions, although in later phases, the deployed teleradiology systems have primarily met the last requirement. Benefits demonstrably shown include decreasing the number of repeated CT scans (decreasing radiation exposure to patients), decreasing the transport of unstable patients to radiology facilities, and improving throughput of patients throughout the health-care system by having accurate diagnostic reports and images available prior to arrival of the patient.

14.6
Iraq (Operation Iraqi Freedom)

The lack of secure DTRS Web servers deployed in the Iraqi theater of operations early in the war led to the loss of patient health-care information in theater, the inability to move critical diagnostic images throughout deployed hospitals (to include the operating room and the emergency room), a lack of greater clinical collaboration with higher echelons of health care, and the lack of a means to electronically transmit and archive patient health-care data/imagery as required by Federal law—the Health Insurance Portability and Accountability Act, passed in 1996.

In June 2004, the Commander, Second Medical Command (MEDCOM), requested that DTRSs be deployed to Baghdad and Balad, Iraq. The request was approved by the Army, and the installation, testing, and training of the equipment to the split 31st CSH in Balad and Baghdad were completed in July 2004. During this trip, the Deputy Commander for Clinical Services, Eighth Medical Brigade in Kuwait, requested teleradiology capabilities for three MTFs in Kuwait. Soon after this request, the 67th CSH requested a DTRS for Mosul, and the Air Force began a separate procurement of a system for its hospital in Ali Al Salaam, Kuwait. On the basis of these requests, systems were procured by the US Army Medical Materiel Agency, located at USAMRMC Fort Detrick, and sent to Kuwait in January 2005.

In January 2005, the 44th MEDCOM requested expansion of the teleradiology storage and distribution functionality for all deployed hospitals in Iraq. This request was completed in March 2005 with the deployment of a DTRS to the Mosul military hospital. Further DTRS deployments in Iraq have taken place as needed since that time, including at the Abu Ghraib and the Buca prison medical facilities.

The greatest use of teleradiology in Iraq has been to forward films of injured soldiers to those hospitals that will be providing follow-on care (Fig. 14.8) [13]. Combat operations in Iraq have provided a steady stream of casualties who have almost all had digital X-rays done in the combat zone. The existing teleradiology system has worked well for basic radiological studies (chest, abdomen, and other plain films), but there are, occasionally, still some problems with the availability of CT scans; the overall impression of the operability of the system by the surgeons using it to treat patients evacuated from the Operation Iraqi Freedom (OIF)/OEF war theater is quite favorable. The newer surgeons at the LRMC report minimal difficulties and have accepted the functional operability of the system as a matter of routine [19]. Once the technology and business practices had matured to the point where clinicians were supportive of the system, the focus of dissatisfaction shifted from complaints about "why are we doing this?" to complaints such as "where are this patient's films?" and

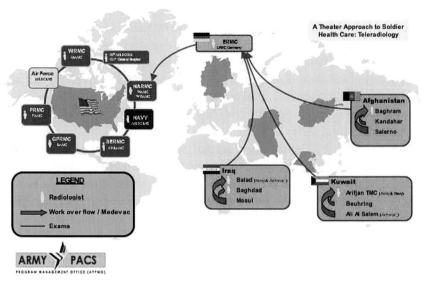

Fig. 14.8. Laydown diagram of Teleradiology in Iraq

"why can't I get them downloaded more quickly?" These issues, in much part, come from the never-ending struggle with the always-present need for more bandwidth. At present, the state has been reached where using teleradiology has become "the way that we do business"; the major remaining issue is how to get enough dedicated bandwidth to Roles 2 and 3 facilities[2] to make the system function better for the users.

Theater teleradiology capabilities have matured significantly over time. As a result, there are three primary use cases that illustrate the use of the transmission of digital images within Iraq as well as to higher echelons of care.

---

[2] "Role" is a NATO term, which describes the capabilities of a specific medical facility. Generally speaking, Role 1 provides advanced trauma life support and routine sick call. Role 2 offers life-saving surgical intervention, although without surgical specialists being assigned. Role 3 is a fully equipped field hospital offering care by clinical specialists, whereas Role 4 is usually found in the national home country and provides a full spectrum of care, including subspecialty and rehabilitative care. The American nomenclature is similar, with the term "Level" being used and with an additional Level 5 being added at the top end of the spectrum.

1. *Trauma/subspecialty consultation*: Images are transmitted from a Role 2 surgical unit or a Role 3 CSH to a Role 3 CSH during an urgent/emergent situation to facilitate rapid decision making regarding surgical treatment, intratheater transfer, or emergency medical evacuation out of theater to a Role 4 or higher facility. An ongoing intratheater example currently includes the urgent need for a general surgeon at a CSH in Baghdad consulting with a physically removed neurosurgeon located at the CSH in Balad (70 km away), regarding a traumatic brain-injured patient's head CT scan, thereby facilitating immediate surgical planning considerations by the general surgeon located in Baghdad.

2. *Routine diagnosis*: Images are transmitted from a Role 2 or 3 CSH to an intratheater Role 3 CSH for the routine diagnostic interpretation of an image by a radiologist. While not urgent, the interpretation of these images may be critical to decisions regarding clinical care, the ability to treat in theater, and/or the need to evacuate the patient out of theater. This comprises the majority of all image transmissions, roughly 75%.

3. *Image archive*: Copies of select images are transmitted from a Role 2 or 3 to a selected Role 4 military medical center (i.e., in Germany or the USA) for long-term archival purposes within 24 h of completion. There is limited storage in theater; therefore, ideally, images should be transferred to central archives. Likewise, patients tend to be transported within this timeframe after a severe injury. Continuity of care is facilitated by the rapid flow of images to a central archive, from which they can be readily retrieved by other medical facilities providing care for the patient.

The network must transmit diagnostic-quality radiology images, as defined in the priority classification table (Table 14.1), across a theater of operations and throughout the global military health system, to support the delivery of prompt medical care for deployed soldiers.

Current bandwidth availability makes effective transmission limited; a recent analysis showed that current transmission times for full CT scans is now measured in hours rather than in minutes. General surgeons, orthopedic surgeons, and other providers in the deployed environment are often focused

Table 14.1. Priority classifications for asynchronous transmission of digital images

Use case	Priority rating	Transmission time
Trauma	1	15 min
Routine diagnosis	2	4 h
Image archive	3	24 h

on obtaining rapid results and making quick management decisions regarding patients who are then quickly transferred to other facilities. With short theater evacuation times (the time a patient may remain in the hospital before evacuation), the focus is on rapid decision making. Although a written report is considered standard of care, the current delay in waiting for a formal written radiology report to become available on the network is frequently not looked at favorably by the deployed surgeons, and they constantly demand faster responses from the system. There are, additionally, two secondary populations who are being treated by the US military in Iraq: local civilians and detainees. Patients in these categories are not being transferred to US facilities outside the theater; their treatment does occasionally require consultation through use of the teleradiology system.

14.7
System Description

1. The Army's DTRS is currently based on the commercially available DICOM-distributed TMED server (Medweb RAQ 5, San Francisco, CA, USA) and provides local image distribution and teleradiology reach-back capability for Roles 2 and 3 medical facilities currently deployed throughout the Iraq and Afghanistan theaters of operation. The Medweb RAQ system allows the collection of all forms of medical imaging data from diagnostic imaging devices such as CT, magnetic resonance imaging, ultrasound, and regular CR X-ray devices over telecommunications networks.
2. Components of the Medweb RAQ system set fielded to the radiology section of deployed CSHs are shown in Table 14.2 (Fig. 14.9).
3. The Medweb server combines the functions of a PACS archive, DICOM Web server, TMED Web server, Ethernet proxy gateway, virtual private network encryption router, and satellite-enhanced DICOM Internet tunnel. Medweb servers are designed to work in pairs to provide 100% redundancy and automatic fail-over operation.
4. The Medweb RAQ is currently being used by CSHs and medical clinics in OIF/OEF. Digital images are assembled on the Medweb server and are made available via a Web interface, forwarded in encrypted format over wide-area network connections, and/or written to CD-ROMs or USB drives, which can be played back on any conventional Windows PC without additional software.

A total of 15 systems have been deployed in Iraq (in Baghdad, Mosul, and Balad) Kuwait, Afghanistan, and Qatar. Put in place by the Army, the technology is shared by all service branches (Fig. 14.10).

Table 14.2. Components of the Medweb RAQ system

Medweb RAQ4 servers with 60 GB hard-disk drive, warm failover software (2)

CD-R/W and USB drive option

Space 60 GB hard-disk drive inside first RAQ

APC Corporation smart uninterruptible power supply 700 2U (switchable power)

Cisco Corporation 24-port 10/100 Ethernet switch (1)

SKB Corporation 24" 1G shock-mount rack case and covers (1)

150 ft Ethernet cables (2)

15 ft Ethernet cables (2)

6 ft Ethernet cables (5)

Spare Cisco Corporation 24-port 10/100 Ethernet switch (1)

Laptop image display computer with auxiliary flat panel display (1)

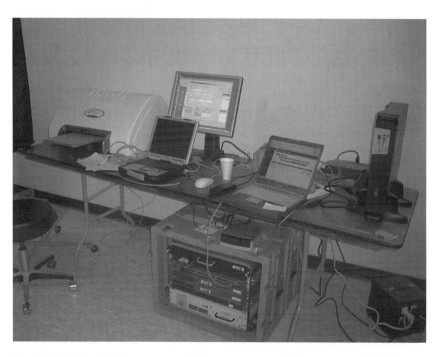

Fig. 14.9. Medweb RAQ system installed in Kuwait, 2005. (Photo courtesy of Medweb)

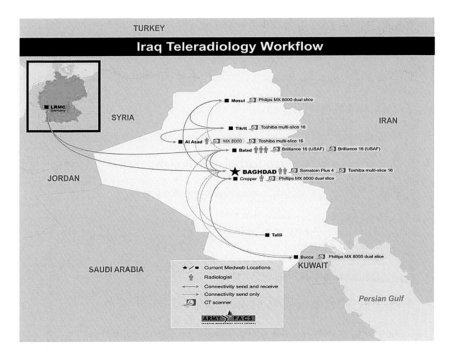

Fig. 14.10. Iraq teleradiology workflow

14.8
Teleradiology in Military Humanitarian Assistance Operations

In addition to combat and peace support operations, the US military also has historically played a significant role in humanitarian and disaster-relief operations [8]. The teleradiology system developed for combat support use also is suitable for use in these operations, although our experience has been that teleradiology plays a lesser role in these operations than in US military combat missions.

The use of digitally sent images taken during humanitarian assistance operations has been described many times in the literature, but there have been few reports of actually using a modern system that is capable of transmitting non-compressed DICOM images. This was accomplished during the 212th MASH medical treatment of casualties following a large earthquake in the Kashmir region of Pakistan in 2005 [14]. During this mission, a robust digital radiology system supported by a Medweb server was deployed and successfully linked to the LRMC DIN-PACS using an MC4 (medical communications for combat casualty care system) Ku band VSAT satellite terminal. The need for radiological consultation was minimal during this mission. A plethora of orthopedic injuries were treated, but outside consultation was not requested by either of the two orthopedic surgeons who were members of the deployed team. In total, three radiology consultations were requested during this relief effort; these were all regarding X-ray images that posed perplexing clinical problems; none of the patients were critically ill, and none of the consultations resulted in a significant change in treatment or notable impact on clinical outcome.

The nature of humanitarian assistance missions does not tend to generate a great need for teleradiology consultation. The "rules of medical engagement," which are used to determine the scope of medical care that is being provided generally, do not require that the US civilian style of medicine be duplicated; this decreases the requirement for the archiving of studies and the necessity for sub-specialty consultation. Also, since the patients are rarely evacuated to US facilities, the need to transfer images to the supporting-level facility is not present.

14.9
Lessons Learned and Issues Still To Be Resolved

In spite of the significant effort expended over the past decades to deploy teleradiology to the field by the US military, some problems remain. While digital imaging technologies are extensively fielded in the OIF/OEF theaters and a telera-diology platform is fully deployed, these capabilities have not been optimized to support medical care. The current systems are not yet being used to their fullest advantage, primarily owing to the telecommunications network deficiencies asso-ciated with the transmission of digital radiographs, advanced TMED applications, and other medical data between NATO Roles 2 and 3 medical units in the OIF/OEF theaters and between those medical units and military treatment facilities worldwide. Medical units are missing the much needed high-speed data network that connects this equipment and platform uniformly between all medical units.

Because of the nonexistence of a standard hospital information system–radiology information system interface and because the pace of clinical work and radiology can be quite rapid, patient demographic information is not always inserted into the DICOM header of the study. This may affect neither the study at the moment nor the use of the study for immediate clinical use, but it does mean that when the study is sent back to the LRMC and the USA, the study may not match the patient's indexed data and will therefore be effectively lost even if it is in the PACS. Thus, many of the studies carried out in theater are not avail-able as a part of the patient's longitudinal patient record.

All of the US military medical services have jointly learned a lot and have developed significant capabilities through combined experiences in Iraq and Afghanistan. Because of network reliability and availability issues, the function of teleradiology in the land-based deployed medical units continues to be primarily for the movement of patient data in support of the medical evacuation process. This in itself has a great positive impact on the individual's health care. When the imaging data are available prior to the arrival of an injured service member, the receiving health-care team can already be prepared to continue care without delay. Given that many of these patients are transferred from one treatment facility to another at least three and as many as six times from the time of injury to the time of discharge from a rehabilitation facility, the reduction in repeat imaging studies and the inherent reduction in radiation exposure also cannot be understated as a benefit. "Jointness" is still a work in progress. The TMED leads are joined and work together as a team, and efforts have resulted in equipping Army-, Navy-, and Air-Force-deployed medical facilities with the same equipment. Full integration of some of the business practices, which will enable true integration of radiology functions across service lines, is still being achieved. We all face the same challenges of bandwidth, money for bandwidth, and bandwidth real estate on the shared lines (we may have military bandwidth available, but not the permission to use it).

There is significant value in having the DICOM server in a Role 2/3 MTF—providing the ability to route images over a LAN to the Emergency Department/operating room/intensive care units, thereby avoiding long walks to the radiology ISO shelter (hardwall shelters, called ISO shelters after the manufacturer, the International Standards Organization) to review films on a laptop! Having the ability to route studies to other intratheater/intertheater MTFs as the casualty goes through the various echelons of care is critical to the continuity of care we are seeking. There is a need to emphasize the reality of our deployed health-care system—we have limited specialists in theater and therefore need to move films to where the specialists are for second opinions—and this requirement goes beyond teleradiology and must address the needs of other subspecialties, e.g., neurosurgery, to review CR and CT scans.

The most significant challenge we face today is summed up in two words—dedicated bandwidth. As noted above, we simply do not have sufficient bandwidth to effectively move images as required to support the clinical practice of radiology in the theater of operations. The fielding of multislice CT scanners and the nature and severity of the injuries we are seeing have exacerbated this problem. Efforts are under way to obtain adequate dedicated bandwidth to enable optimum usage of this capability. Development of a Department of Defense (DoD) medical-dedicated network will solve most of the interoperability challenges we currently face and will greatly facilitate the movement of images intratheater and intertheater.

In Iraq, digital radiographs are currently being transported across a combination of low-bandwidth networks to include, but not limited to, VSAT and local military-provided communication links. These networks were not designed to handle the file size (10–120 MB) or the volume of images being generated in theater by CR. Further, the management of these networks is divided among various groups, making the management and allocation of bandwidth more complex.

In July 2007, a study was conducted in Iraq to prove the concept that a committed information rate (CIR)—or dedicated bandwidth—could improve network performance and meet medical requirements. Initial testing revealed that a CIR of 300 kbps up/768 kbps down could meet the requirement to move any image within the 15-min threshold set for trauma patients. Details of this study are not currently available for publication, but the study demonstrated that clinical gains in digital image transmission can be made with better bandwidth management and allocation. Efforts are currently under way to gain military support for the concept of dedicated bandwidth to support the medical requirements.

The desired capabilities of the proposed dedicated medical system are detailed below.

The network must be capable of transmitting, between Role 3 facilities (intratheater), diagnostic-quality radiology images up to 120 MB in file size within 15 min, while simultaneously permitting other medical applications, including video teleconferencing, to occur without network degradation. This capability should also be available between any Role 3 facility and the LRMC and should leverage all current and planned telecommunications network upgrades.

1. *Performance*: The network must transmit diagnostic-quality radiology images, as defined in the priority classification table (Table 14.1), across a theater of operations and the global military health system, to support the delivery of prompt medical care for deployed soldiers.
2. *Capacity*: The network must support the concurrent utilization of four main categories of medical applications for purposes of delivering high-quality medical care in the field: (1) radiology, (2) video teleconferencing, (3) Theater Medical Information Program (TMIP) suites, and (4) Web-based applications.
3. *Distribution*: The desired system must provide a ubiquitous network linking all Roles 2 and 3 MTFs to each other and all Role 3 CSHs to the LRMC, to allow the seamless flow of medical data and images to and from all nodes on the network in a theater of operations.

In addition to moving imagery from one point to another within the hospital, the DTRS servers provide a means of storing medical imagery and patient information for long-term retrieval and forwarding diagnostic information on patients evacuated to higher echelons of health care outside theater, providing a more complete medical record of injury and subsequent care. Beneficial to the long-term care of soldiers, the DTRS servers inherently support the AMEDD goal in providing an electronic medical record that remains with the soldier long after leaving the battlefield.

14.10
Summary/Discussion

Across the world, the US military medical services are today approximately 90% digital with respect to digital radiology [20]. A variety of different PACS from different vendors have been installed throughout the services at a cost of over $600 million. These systems all use the DICOM standard as their imaging format and are thus able to transfer images and reports as needed to both deployed and fixed military health-care facilities. This system remains a bit awkward at present and requires a number of functional workarounds, but, in spite of these deficiencies, several hundred thousand images are transferred between facilities every year for remote interpretation, reporting, subspecialty consultation, and archiving, and this figure continues to grow.

The military health system's AHLTA longitudinal health record and the theater electronic health record are in the process of building a more coherent integration of medical and dental imaging and associated reporting/storage capabilities into the electronic health record to create a comprehensive and continuous multimedia longitudinal electronic medical record, which begins in the deployed situation and extends back into the garrison health-care system. This system will provide enhanced quality of care through its improvement of medical handoff of the care of medical evacuees and its support for day-to-day care for service members and their families. Part of the global strategy of the military health system is to have medical record information of all types readily available to the veterans affairs (VA) health-care providers upon transition of service members to the VA's health-care system.

This effort at improved integration began with funded pilot projects in financial years 2006 and 2007. It will continue to be supported in the financial year 2008 and 2009 DoD budgets. An additional effort is ongoing to enhance existing business process relationships between partner VA hospitals and associated DoD and civilian medical institutions, to ensure that our service members' medical information is accessible when needed and that these systems are interoperable to the greatest degree possible. To accomplish this goal, the military has chartered the PACS Joint Services Working Group (JSWG) to address medical imaging integration needs and to champion coherent changes. To date, the PACS JSWG members have been successful in bringing DoD and the VA health-care delivery systems closer together from an imaging and interoperability perspective. Further, the VA has looked carefully at the DoD's successful deployed teleradiology systems, in order to support their goal of bringing the VA and DoD health-care systems closer together to support the increasingly dynamic workflows, which are necessary between VA facilities and with the DoD, if we are to provide optimum support to our beneficiaries. The military and the VA are in agreement that we must continue to work together to support our shared health-care populations with better and more efficient health-care processes. This, in turn, will help us provide the best possible standard of care to our beneficiaries and reduce the per capita costs of health care. It is all about quality and throughput.

14.11
The Future of Military Radiology

The US military medical services have effectively migrated to digital radiology technology and workflows and now are approximately 90% digital in their radiology operations, both in the garrison and in the field. All DoD medical centers have PACS and teleradiology, and the ongoing installation of digital radiology at all of our smaller medical facilities ensures that almost every small medical facility will soon be connected to a larger center for radiology diagnosis.

Whether in a deployed setting or in a garrison, teleradiology has become the way we do business in the US military. Although there are still areas in which we need to make improvements, we currently have what we consider to be the most effective and most widespread teleradiology system in the world. We have made it effective by applying current peacetime radiology business practices and processes to the deployed environment. It is becoming more and more apparent that "teleradiology" is a term that is destined to be eliminated, as in today's military "teleradiology" and "radiology" are one and the same. The system works effectively at present, since it is simply creating a mirror image of our usual medical business processes.

We believe that the prefix "tele" in "teleradiology" will soon be a term of the past, as the system is evolving toward the goal of a "vendor-neutral" network, which will provide totally seamless integration of the multiple sources of care. The future for the word "teleradiology" is retirement. Once the network functionality and bandwidth availability problems are overcome, the practice of radiology across the world will be no different from the practice within a medical facility.

Summary

- Use of radiography in the field has been one of the greatest medical contributions to the recovery of a wounded soldier.
- Developments in radiology in the US military started after the Vietnam War and now deployable digital radiography is increasingly in use with many armed forces.

- The teleradiology system developed for combat support use is also suitable in humanitarian and disaster-relief operations performed by armed forces.
- Teleradiology application to military medical services has its limitations. However, once the network functionality and bandwidth availability problems are overcome, the practice of radiology across the world will be no different from that within a medical facility.

References

1. Abbott FC (1899) Surgery in the Graeco-Turkish War. Lancet 80:80–83
2. Abbott FC (1899) Surgery in the Graeco-Turkish War. Lancet 80:133–134
3. Alvaro G (1964) The practical benefits to surgery of Röntgen's discovery (diagnostic results in the location of bullets in wounded soldiers from Africa). In: Bruwer AJ (ed) Classic descriptions in diagnostic roentgenology, vol. 2. Thomas, Springfield, pp 1318–1323
4. Battersby J (1899) The present condition of the Roentgen rays in military surgery. Arch Roentgen Ray 3:74–80, 89–91
5. Beevor WC (1898) The working of the Roentgen ray in warfare. J R United Serv Inst 42:1152–1170
6. Borden WC (1900) The use of the Röntgen ray by the Medical Department of the United States Army in the war with Spain (1898). Government Printing Office, Washington, DC
7. Crowther JB, Poropatich RK (1995) Telemedicine in the U.S. Army: case reports from Somalia and Croatia. Telemedicine 1:73–80
8. Foster GM (1983) The demands of humanity: Army medical disaster relief. Center of Military History, Washington
9. Gower DW, Phillips RA, Smith SD, Gallego J, Forkner E, Cooke M (1997) Bosnia telemedicine evaluation final report (USAMEDDBD Project 2-96), US Army Medical Department Center and School, Fort Sam Houston
10. Harcke HT, Statler JD, Montilla J (2006) Radiology in a hostile environment—experience in Afghanistan. Mil Med 171(3):194–199
11. Johnston GC (1923–1929) Division of roentgenology. In: War Department, Surgeon General's Office. The Medical Department of the United States Army in the World War, vol. 1. Government Printing Office, Washington, pp 465–473
12. Küttner H (1898) The importance of Roentgen rays in war surgery based on experience in the Greco-Turkish war of 1897. Beitr Klin Chir 20:167–230
13. Lam D, MacKenzie C (2005) Human and organizational factors affecting telemedicine utilization within U.S. Military Forces in Europe. Telemed J E-Health 11(1):51–59
14. Lam D, Meade K (2007) A deployable telemedicine capability in support of humanitarian operations. Telemed E-Health 13(3):331–340
15. Levine BA, Cleary K, Mun SK (1998) Lessons learned from the DEPRAD deployment. PACMEDTEK Symposium, Honolulu Hawaii
16. Lyche DK, de Treville RE, Norton GS, Leckie RG (1994) Medical diagnostic imaging support early experience and efficacy of wide-area intercontinental teleradiology. Proc SPIE 2165:271–282

17. Lyche DK, Weiser JC, Romlein J, Goeringer F, Scotti S (1995) PACS and teleradiology in the Department of Defense. In: Eighth IEEE symposium on computer-based medical systems (CBMS'95). Los Alamitos, Calif. : IEEE Computer Society Press
18. Mun SK, Levine BA, Cleary K, Dai H (1998) Deployable teleradiology and telemedicine for the US military. Computer Methods and Programs in Biomedicine, Elsevier Science Ireland LTD., 57:21–27
19. Parsons DM, Kim Y (1994) Quality control assessment for the medical diagnostic imaging support (MDIS) system's display monitors. Proc SPIE 2164:186–197
20. Poropatich R, Detreville R, Lappan C, Barrigan C (2006) The U.S. Army Telemedicine program: general overview and current status in Southwest Asia. Telemed E-Health 12(4):396–408
21. Röntgen WC (1895) Ueber eine neue Art von Strahlen (vorläufige Mittheilung). Ber Phys Med Ges Wurzbg 132–141

15

Teleradiology for Traumatic Brain Injury Management

CORRADO IACCARINO, ARMANDO RAPANA', CHRISTIAN COMPAGNONE, FERNANDA TAGLIAFERRI, and FRANCO SERVADEI

Abstract Teleradiology experiences from workstation to wireless technology and discrepancies from an "ideal world" of guidelines and a "real world" of medical practice are detailed. The real predictive value of Glasgow Coma Scale admission for the outcome of brain-injured patients and differences regarding the outcome of traumatic brain injury patients treated with or without neurosurgical facilities are outlined. Also examined is how to detect the computed tomography evolution before the neurologic change and the application of guidelines with area protocol and "hub and spoke" systems is discussed.

15.1
Background Information

The selection of patients admitted to the neurosurgical center is usually based on a telephonic consultation (TC) with the neurosurgeon on duty. In many neurosurgical units, it is available as teleradiology (TR) where the TC is integrated with the direct view of each patient's computed tomography (CT) scans via image transmission. Guidelines for the management of severe traumatic brain injury (TBI) patients have been published both in the USA [7, 10] and in Europe [27]. Unfortunately, none of these guidelines, except in part those from Italy (Table 15.1) [44], contain clear statements about which patients should be admitted to a neurosurgical center.

When an interaction occurs between a primary-care physician at one site and a specialist at another, the accuracy of information exchange during a TC depends on the reliability and completeness of the information received from referral hospitals [51] and the experience of the referring physician [31, 63]. The use of TR reduces the incidence of unnecessary transfer and adverse effects occurring during transfer [18], when there are guidelines and information technology is a well-established part of the physician's experience. This dual-authority system within health-care organizations creates opportunities for potential conflicts in telemedicine-related decisions.

Table 15.1. Italian guidelines for the treatment of traumatic brain injury patients: summary on transfer of comatose patients [44]

First scenario	At the scene of an accident, a comatose patient is not yet stable despite all therapeutic efforts. The patient must be taken to the nearest hospital with a general surgery department, an ICU, and a radiology department with full X-ray and ultrasound diagnostic facilities. Brain CT scans may be postponed until respiratory and circulatory stabilities are achieved. The neurosurgical department should anyway be informed so as to be ready to admit the stabilized patient
Second scenario	At the scene of an accident, a comatose patient has stable circulation and respiration. Whenever direct access to a neurosurgical center is not feasible, the patient must be admitted to a hospital providing, at least, the following:
	– An ICU that can ensure ventilatory assistance, invasive arterial monitoring, serial blood gas analysis, hourly neurological assessment (GCS and pupils), 24 h medical staff, and, at least, one nurse to every two patients – 24 h CT scan facilities and immediate interpretation
	On admission the following are indispensable:
	– Continuation and optimization of intensive care – Diagnostic definition of brain injury (brain scan) and cervical spine (including the cervicodorsal junction), within 3 h of injury – Diagnosis of concomitant lesions (X-ray of the chest and pelvis and abdominal ultrasonography) – Neurosurgical consultation, either directly or by transmission of images and clinical information, to establish whether transfer is urgent or can be planned subsequently
Third scenario	At the scene of an accident or during transport to the first hospital, a comatose patient presents with worsening of the GCS, progressive papillary alterations, and/or motor signs of cerebral coning. The patient must be taken to the nearest neurosurgical center since the risk of a surgical intracranial hematoma is extremely high

ICU intensive care unit, *CT* computed tomography, *CGS* Glasgow Coma Scale

The quality of the imaging, the feasibility of sharing pictures, and software play an important role in the efficacy of TR. The technological knowledge should be rapidly upgraded in the cultural background within health-care organizations.

The DICOM standard represents the only established technical protocol, while many workstations for telemedicine are available with different software

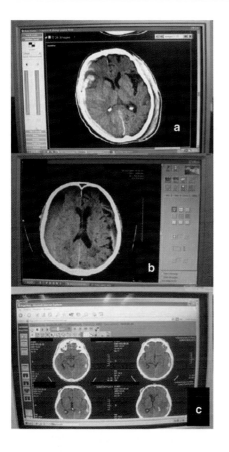

Fig. 15.1. In the "Hub & Spoke" neurosurgical center of Parma and Reggio Emilia (Italy), there are three different types of software for telemedicine (**a–c**) for three different teleradiology (TR) workstations. Each workstation is connected to a server of a different radiology unit of any general hospital (GH) in a specific geographical area. Each peripheral server is connected to other smaller radiology units of other hospitals

(Fig. 15.1). Moreover, the telemedicine installations can employ different types of Internet connections, from ADSL lines to broadband connections of up to 1 GB/s.

An important event in telecounseling may be the introduction of interactive video teleconferencing systems into the health-care environment-integrated health-care systems [32]. With this integrated technology, it is possible to perform videocounseling (VC): patients and any relevant radiological images could be visualized at the same time, using the real-time interactive videoconferencing equipment.

Whether VC is a significant improvement with respect to TR is still being debated. Wong et al. [65], in a 3-year period, recruited 710 patients in a teaching hospital which served a population of 1.5 million. Within each brain disease category (head injury, hemorrhages, and miscellaneous), patients were further randomized through use of double-sealed envelopes into TC, TR, and VC categories. The authors concluded that the use of TR and VC achieved an unequivocally better diagnostic accuracy than use of TC alone. However, this improvement failed to translate into benefits in clinical outcomes or cost-effectiveness. It is possible that the favorable impact of VC over TR is overshadowed by the importance of TR over conventional TC.

The referral protocol of the patients is another important aspect of TR, but the development of guidelines depends on the different scenarios where TR could be applied. How can we compare a province on the east coast of South Africa, with a population of about eight million, and only one public neurosurgical hospital (NH) [73], with a large district general hospital (GH) with a tertiary neurosurgical center and a population of 1.5 million in Hong Kong, China [65], or an Italian region of the northeast, with a population of about one million, with five major hospitals computer-linked [51] with the neurosurgical center? Obviously, in these different locations there are different clinical, economical, and political aspects that can influence the management of TBI.

Anyway, the combination of TR and guidelines for head injury management could allow, in such different areas, a better selection of patients for referral for neurosurgery.

15.2
Global Experience

The global experience is favorable to TR in head injury management. The conclusions about the benefits, the related reduction of costs, and the more rational use of resources are reported in most papers about TR and TBI.

In several recent papers, some discrepancies are reported from an "ideal world" of medical and surgical guidelines and the "real world" of the medical practice [6, 60, 62] in TBI management. Recent appraisals of the early management of patients with TBI from the Scottish Intercollegiate Guidelines Network [47], the Royal College of Paediatrics and Child Health, and the National Institute for Clinical Excellence [35] all recommend that the "transfer of a child to a specialist neurosurgical unit should be undertaken by staff experienced in the transfer of critically ill children—i.e, a (Regional) Paediatric Transfer Team." After a 12-month audit of emergency access to all specialist neurosurgical and intensive care services, the UK Paediatric Brain Injury Study Group and the Paediatric Intensive Care Society Study Group concluded that the recommendation to use specialist regional pediatric transfer teams delays rather than expedites the emergency service [58].

Undoubtedly, a highly technological network, where clinical and neurodiagnostic information of TBI patients can be quickly shared between physicians and specialists, represents a more rational use of resources than a simple phone connection. The "hot question" now is well summarized in a paper by Patel et al. [40]: How can we improve the management of TBI patients when a significant number of cases are not admitted to NHs? Furthermore, what differences do we see about the outcome of TBI patients treated with or without neurosurgical facilities [51, 53, 62]?

It is very difficult to evaluate the real efficacy of TR on the outcome of TBI patients owing to the lack of any clinical and radiological follow-up for patients primarily not admitted to a neurosurgery unit [51]. Moreover, the efficiency of TR depends on clinical, logistic, and technical aspects of the health-care system.

Ashkenazi et al.[2] recently showed that in a rural level 2 trauma center without neurosurgical capacity, a trauma team, neurosurgical consultation, and TR are the fundamental requisites to treat just selective head-injured patients with a pathological CT scan. They also concluded that it was necessary to carefully reevaluate the currently existing transfer criteria.

In 2004, Poca et al. [43] reported the use of a teleradiological link between a neurosurgical center and a GH in Spain. The authors concluded that the use of TR in the daily management of head-injured patients provides clear benefits, leads to a more rational use of resources, and reduces costs. Nevertheless, what is pinpointed in this report is how the effectiveness of the system depends more on the infrastructure of the health system in each geographical area than on sophisticated telemedicine systems.

To reduce the negative impact of a too-elongated learning curve of the use of telemedicine systems on the efficiency of TR, several authors proposed a wireless technology with the use of commercial tools such as mobile phones or a personal digital assistant (PDA).

During the past 10 years, Yamamoto et al. [68–72] showed how wireless and compression imaging technologies could facilitate telemedicine.

In 2003, Yamada et al. [67] first reported the transmission of photographed CT scans with the use of a mobile phone, with a 110,000-pixel digital camera and a built-in thin-film transistor liquid crystal display (LCD) that uses up to 65,536 colors. The display size was $31 \times 30\,mm^2$. The images were 120×128 pixel JPEG files. The medical images photographed by the digital camera were taken from the computer screen, or from the light box, and then attached to a mobile phone e-mail message.

Two years later, Kim et al. [21] proposed the use of a PDA phone with a built-in camera, supporting various image resolutions. The images were displayed on the sender and receiver PDA 240×320 pixels TFT LCD screen. Data transmission used a wireless high-bandwidth network (CDMA1_EVDO) interface wireless local-area network card for wireless communication. The network had a maximum transfer rate of $2\,Mbit/s$ for the downlink and $153\,kbit/s$ for the uplink. They concluded that a minimum of 640 × 480 image resolution for CT and MRI and 1,024 × 768 image resolution for angiography appeared to offer the best compromise for making urgent medical decisions. In 2007, Kim et al. [22] showed the same system with the PDA sender and a PC-based picture archiving and communication system terminal linked with Bluetooth-interfaced local wireless.

In 2007, Ng et al. [36] reported a system analogous to that of Yamada et al. [67] for photographing CT/MRI images with a mobile phone with a video graphics array camera, sending the images by multimedia messaging service (MMS) mobile phone technology. All consultants had personal mobile phones that were MMS-enabled, allowing them to access the images from anywhere without the need for a workstation (TR or Internet) to make a clinical decision.

Mobile TR could be a practical solution in rural areas, in developing countries with a few and distant neurosurgical facilities, or in geographical areas with dispersed population nuclei such as archipelagos, where the lack of neurosurgical expertise and the reduced economical resources pose a significant problem.

Compared with the costly TR equipment, with a static workstation to view incoming images that requires sophisticated training and skill to operate, the mobile-phone method could be adequately useful in industrialized areas too.

There are some problems related to this kind of transmission. The static images do not allow one to modify the images by adjusting the window level or rapidly scrolling the images. Another limit is the key image selection by the triaging health-care professional. The imaging quality is anyway adequate for an accurate diagnosis and subsequent initiation of treatment in a timely fashion, as reported in further studies [23, 42]. To avoid any bias of interpretation, the entire CT scan study should be sent. In 2004, Yaghmai et al. [66] described a simple technique for transmission of a complete set of cranial CT images to a commercially available wireless PDA for remote TR consultation. The images were retrieved, decompressed, and transmitted to a remote radiologist's wireless PDA with mobile-phone capability. The entire procedure (including image capture, transmission, and review) took approximately 11.5 min.

For this kind of mobile TR, it could be useful to propose a protocol of image selection where the most reliable CT findings for a brain injury are detectable. We probably need to see the status of basal cisterns, the most cranial and caudal scans where a mass lesion is visible, the scans with the maximum mass effect, or the greater shift of midline.

In conclusion, we believe that, owing to the abovementioned limitation, JPEG image transmission, with MMS or e-mail (Fig. 15.2), should be limited to areas where more comprehensive systems cannot be used.

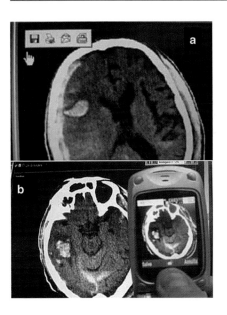

Fig. 15.2. JPEG TR system: **a** directly from the TR workstation it is possible to send a JPEG file by e-mail or to save it on an external drive and **b** with a mobile phone with a built-in camera it is possible to send a multimedia messaging service message with the chosen computed tomography (CT) scan

15.3
Education and Training

The reasons for many physicians' underuse of the TR network are numerous: lack of information, interest or familiarity with the technology; no contact with the referring physicians; and delays in obtaining a reply for nonemergency cases. In addition, there is the lack of financial recognition for the responding physician. These factors correspond to the many organizational barriers to the development of TR that have been described in the literature [13, 24, 28, 41, 45, 55]. Better information should be given to the professionals concerned, and regular training is required. From a technical viewpoint, the number of workstations for sending and receiving transmissions should be increased, and data transmission through a regional network server should be offered.

The appropriate decision for a secondary transfer relies on the quality of the relationships between physicians in the community and those in the NHs [6]. The fate of head-injured patients depends initially on the "neurosurgical qualification" of the primary care. Although image information plays an important role, the neurological findings, physical data, anamnesis, and recent disease history are mandatory to complete the priority list to decide on the management of a patient.

15.3.1
Glasgow Coma Scale Value

In 2001, Schuhmann et al. [46], in Hanover, reported over a 1-year period, in a database of 1,819 entries, an incidence of patients requiring neurosurgical acute care of 75–115 per 100,000 inhabitants per year. Only 30% of patients came directly via the emergency room. In the face of such logistic problems, it is a fundamental necessity that general surgeons triage head-injured patients on the basis of the Glasgow Coma Scale (GCS) and CT scan findings.

Unfortunately, the real predictive value of GCS admission for the outcome of brain-injured patients is nowadays under discussion. In fact, most TBI patients in Europe are often intubated, ventilated, and sedated at the scene of the injury and arrive at the hospitals in a clinical state where the GCS is no longer accurate. A large number of patients were admitted to peripheral hospitals with a GCS of 3, but the outcome of these patients was far better than the outcome of similar patients admitted to the centralized hospital. The GCS, especially GCS 3, in peripheral hospitals may not be reliable [3, 62].

In 2007, Zulu et al. [73] reported that the outcome of TBI patients is determined primarily by the GCS on presentation, rather than the delay before surgery. These considerations could be biased by the low incidence of severe head injuries in this study. Prolonged injury-to-hospital times are not uncommon in South Africa, and those who require urgent neurosurgical intervention for a mass lesion would not survive before reaching a hospital.

The GCS does not entirely allow us to classify patients' risk of radiological deterioration. Therefore, repeat CT in the presence of lesions with high risk of evolution (extradural hematomas; contusions; traumatic subarachnoid hemorrhage, tSAH; etc.) is mandatory within 6–12 h from the first CT scan [49].

Following the publication of the CT classification of Marshall et al. [29], a CT criterion such as a hematoma volume over 25 cm^3 was considered as the "prevailing" indication for evacuation of posttraumatic hematomas.

With a population of about eight million, only one neurosurgical unit, and six general surgical units [73], it is easy to understand how the recommendations to perform a CT scan or to transfer patients to a rare and precious neurosurgical bed should be restrictive and essential. Patients with intracranial abnormalities underwent surgery when they fulfilled one or more of the following criteria: size of lesion of more than 30 cm^2, midline shift of more than 10 mm, and effacement of the ipsilateral ventricle [73]. Conversely, the criteria indicating the performance of a semielective CT scan during hospitalization include any deterioration in the level of consciousness, development of neurological deficit, or failure of improvement of the GCS for more than 48 h, even in the absence of a fracture or focal signs. In this way, the concept of "neuroworsening" is necessarily wider than the NICE recommendations available at http://www.nice.org.uk.

In the series of Marshall et al., patients with evacuated mass lesions (larger than 25 cm^3) had a favorable outcome of 23%, compared with an outcome of 11% in patients with nonevacuated mass lesions. Unfortunately, data from the European Brain Injury Consortium evaluating a series of 724 patients with moderate to severe TBI did not confirm this finding. The rate of favorable outcomes was 45% in patients with evacuated mass lesions, compared with 42% in patients with nonevacuated mass lesions [49]. This is not surprising: surgical indications are, in fact, related to many factors, including the clinical status, the occurrence of clinical deterioration, and CT parameters like the lesion volume but also the amount of midline shift and cistern compression and the lesion location [9].

In spite of the absence of a class I paper, guidelines have been published [9] about surgical management of TBI. A conservative management of selected cases is possible but only when patients with uncertain surgical indications are admitted to neurosurgical centers. The hematomas may evolve over time, and the indication for surgery is a dynamic process, which can also change over time. This implies, at least in Europe, a new discussion about patients' centralization.

15.3.2
GH Versus NH

A recent British paper [40] demonstrated worse outcomes in TBI patients admitted to nonneurosurgical centers in the UK. Data prospectively collected from the Trauma Audit & Research Network (https://www.tarn.ac.uk/) were studied to compare mortality in polytrauma patients (with and without head injury) and in TBI patients admitted to GHs and NHs. Patients with head injury had a tenfold higher mortality, and patients admitted to nonneurosurgical centers had a 2.15-fold increase in the odds of death adjusted for case mix; similar data were published for Italy [51, 53]. The first duty of a neurosurgeon is to evaluate and select patients for admission to specialized centers, even with modern telemedicine systems [51]. This "selection" must contain all possible surgical candidates. The lesson learned recently is that neither a good clinical status on admission nor a small hematoma seen on the first CT scan obtained can exclude subsequent surgical indications [53].

In an ideal world, we would devote enough resources for the best possible treatment of all TBI patients. In the real world, this does not happen even in the richest of Western countries [17]. Recently, a new "factor" appeared to influence the transfer decision.

North American researchers have reported that payer status of the injured patient is an important factor for admission to a level I trauma center [34]. This factor is called an "unspoken triage criterion," since it is not reported in most studies of trauma management. In Europe, we have a similar "unspoken" triage criterion: patient age.

An Italian report [62] compared clinical features and outcomes in two series of severe TBI patients: those admitted to a NH and those admitted to a GH. For patients admitted to the NH, age, CT Marshall EBIC-modified [49] classification (Table 15.2), and GCS were predictors of a favorable outcome, while for patients treated in GHs, CT classification, gender, and age were predictors of a favorable outcome. It was interesting to note that the features of patients treated in centralized NHs versus those treated in GHs were different. Patients treated in NHs were younger, more frequently male; the admission GCS was higher; and the CT classification was different (Table 15.3).

Age has been reported to be the only significant factor in predicting the transfer of patients to NHs in telemedicine systems [51]. Patients older than 65 years were less likely to be transferred to NHs, but when they reached

Table 15.2. CT classification according to Marshall et al. [29], slightly modified according to the EBIC core data survey [51]

Type	Subtype	Cisterns	Shift (mm)	Description
I: Normal CT		Present	0	Intracranial abnormality not visible on CT scan
II: Diffuse injury	(a) Only (b) ≥2 unilateral lesions (c) Bilateral	Present	0–5	Lesion present, but no high- or mixed-density lesion >25 cm³. May include bone fragment and foreign bodies
III: Diffuse injury + swelling		Compressed or absent	0–5	Lesion present, but no high- or mixed-density lesion >25 cm³
IV: Diffuse injury + shift		Compressed or absent	>5	Lesion present, but no high- or mixed-density lesion >25 cm³
V: Evacuated mass lesion	(a) Extradural (b) Subdural (c) Intracerebral (d) ≥2 lesions	Any lesion surgically evacuated		
VI: Nonevacuated mass lesion	(a) Extradural (b) Subdural (c) Intracerebral (d) ≥2 lesions	High- or mixed-density lesion >25 cm³, not surgically evacuated		

Table 15.3. Demographic, clinical, and radiological characteristics of neurosurgical hospital (*NH*) and general hospital (*GH*) study populations [62]

		NH	GH
Gender	Male	264 (75.6%)	118 (60.5%)
	Female	85 (24.4%)	77 (39.5%)
Age	Average	38.5	57
	Median	28	75
GCS	Median on admission	6	3
CT classification	DI I 1 (normal CT)	35 (10.0%)	4 (2.3%)
	DI II 2 (diffuse injury)	236 (67.6%)	96 (54.2%)
	DI III 3 (diffuse injury with compression)	42 (12.0%)	18 (10.2%)
	DI IV 4 (diffuse injury with shift)	28 (8.0%)	35 (19.8%)
	NEML 6 (nonevacuated mass lesion)	8 (2.3%)	24 (13.6%)
Outcome	Unfavorable	132 (37.8%)	109 (55.9%)
	Favorable	217 (62.2%)	86 (44.1%)

a neurosurgical unit the rate of surgical intervention was similar to that of younger patients [33]. In this report, the decision to transfer trauma patients to NHs appears to favor younger patients. Age is a powerful predictor of poor outcomes, as reported in 2003 by Hukkelhoven et al. [19], in an analysis of more than 5,000 patients, or in a study of Oertel et al. [37] in 2002, where the older patients were more likely to have a progression than younger patients with a *p* value of 0.01, adjusted from logistic regression analysis. Nevertheless, there are no published guidelines that give specific age limits for patient transfer [7, 27, 44].

The finding of the difference in gender between peripheral and central hospitals is another new different finding but can be explained. Although the incidence of head injury is higher in younger men, elderly TBI patients are more equally distributed between men and women, with a slightly higher female incidence over the age of 70 years [57]. Therefore, in peripheral hospitals, the number of women with TBI admitted is more higher.

In 2003, Farin et al. [16] showed that in peripheral hospitals outcomes were worse in women, with an increased incidence of brain swelling, similar to the Italian report [62].

15.3.3
CT Evolution

In 2007, Brown et al. [5] prospectively followed almost 300 patients with blunt trauma who had an initially abnormal head on CT. They confirmed what other reports [56] have documented: patients with mild head injury and no neurologic change do not need routine repeat imaging of their head. In the 27% of CT progression, there was no need of any medical or surgical intervention. Conversely, in this series as in other reports [61], all mildly injured patients requiring intervention had clinical deterioration preceding repeat head CT.

It is more difficult to find any strong conclusions regarding the patients with moderate head injury. From literature data, a clear conclusion that can be drawn with regard to patients with moderate and severe head injury is that they should undergo a repeat CT scan after clinical deterioration. Cerebral contusions have a 51% incidence of evolution in the first hours after injury [37]. Lobato et al. [26] reported, in 56 severe head injury patients, new contusion in 26.8% of the patients, growing of previous contusion in 68.2%, or previous extra-axial hematoma in 10.7% of the patients.

In the discussion of the report of Brown et al., Alex B. Valadka emphasized the role of the routine repeat head scanning for patients who may not have yet demonstrated clinical deterioration. He remembers his clinical experience with patients in whom he did an intervention based on a routine scan before those patients got sick.

How can one detect CT evolution before the neurologic change? Kaups et al. [20] identified coagulopathy, hypotension, and depressed GCS score as risk factors for progression of injury. Likewise, Velmahos et al. [61] found older age, lower GCS score, and the presence of multiple lesions on CT scan to be independent risk factors of radiographic progression. In a review of Wang et al. [64], coagulopathy and a higher injury severity scale were the most frequently identified risk factors for progression of injury.

More recently, Beaumont and Gennarelli [4] stated that age, sex, or injury severity have less influence than the presence of edema surrounding the area of hemorrhagic products on first the CT.

The presence of contusions at admission identifies a population at high risk of progression [12]. The neuronal degeneration may be a delayed process occurring on the first to third days after injury owing to a significant release of cytotoxic excitatory amino acids in hemorrhagic contusions [8]. Several recent studies have examined the progression of intraparenchymal contusions and hematomas (IPHs) [37, 38, 39, 48]. In 2006, Chang et al. [11] enrolled 113 patients with mild (46%), moderate (26%), and severe (28%) brain injuries in a retrospective database. They observed nearly 40% of progression on to larger lesions, 11% by 2–5 cm^3 and 15% by more than 5 cm^3. The authors did not find any single parameter as an accurate predictor of growth of IPHs, but they concluded that patients with concurrent tSAH or subdural hematoma and large initial size need to be monitored carefully. Small IPHs tended to remain stable, whereas larger IPHs were not only more likely to progress but also more likely to grow by larger amounts.

Chieregato et al. [12] in a retrospective study revealed significant progression on the CT scan in 42.2% of 141 patients with brain contusion and subarachnoid hemorrhage, presenting mild (59.6%), moderate (14.9%), and severe (25.5%) brain injury. In this study, the doubling of one diameter of the contusion was defined as a sign of clear progression, while a significant progression was defined as a progressive change in the Marshall classification, as suggested by Lobato et al. [25] and later confirmed by the EBIC study [49]. In a population of 142 head-injured patients (who on average underwent their first CT scan within 2 h of injury), Oertel et al. [37] observed a progressive hemorrhage on the second CT scan in 42% of all patients and in 49% of patients who underwent their first CT scan within 2 h of injury. The rates of hemorrhagic progression for IPHs, epidural hematoma, subdural hematoma, and tSAH were 51, 22, 11, and 17%, respectively.

The cytotoxic substances of the hemorrhagic contusions are also released into the extracellular space when the subarachnoid blood enters the brain through the damaged pia or arachnoid membrane [30]. This explains why the combination of tSAH and brain contusions on an admission CT scan identifies patients at the highest risk of evolving brain damage [1, 12, 15, 50, 54].

There is a strong, highly statistically significant association between the presence of tSAH and poor outcomes related to the severity of the initial mechanical damage, rather than to the effects of delayed vasospasm and secondary ischemic brain damage [52]. Furthermore, tSAH may primarily be an early indicator of evolving brain injury (Figs. 15.3, 15.4).

Fainardi et al. [15] evaluated the time course of the worst CT scan in serial CT studies to determine the timing of repeat CT in a population of tSAH patients. In all, 42.6% of the patients were classified as having mild, 31.9% as moderate, and 25.5% as severe head injury. The author found that the "worst CT examination" corresponded to the first CT scan in 41.1% of cases, whereas in 58.9% patients it was obtained as a subsequent CT study. In the last subset of patients, the median time from trauma to the "worst CT scan" was 29.3 h. In addition, a "significant CT evolution" with a change in the Marshall EBIC-modified classification was found in 26.9% patients with tSAH, with a trend toward a higher risk of evolution in patients with the presence of tSAH over the cerebral convexities. Therefore, a second CT scan should be repeated at

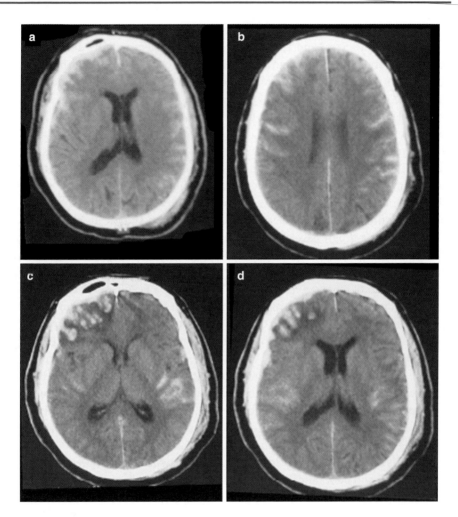

Fig. 15.3. A 66-year-old patient involved in a road traffic accident. Admission Glasgow Coma Scale (GCS) score of 13. **a, b** Initial CT scan, 90 min after injury, shows diffuse bilateral traumatic subarachnoid hemorrhage (tSAH) localized in the sulci on the brain vault and a small right frontal subdural hematoma. **c, d** CT scans performed 8 h later show right frontal progressive parenchymal damage. (From [12])

12–24 h, whereas a third CT scan may be rescheduled between 24 and 48 h after the initial CT scan.

Conversely, in 268 patients younger than 18 years of age, Durham et al. [14] found no significantly increased risk for patients with subarachnoid hemorrhage.

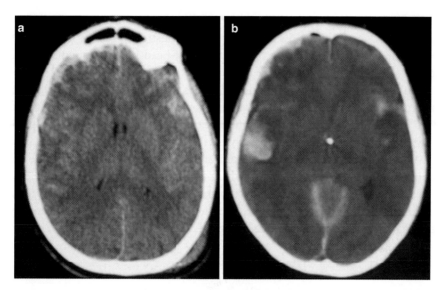

Fig. 15.4. A 52-year-old patient involved in a road traffic accident. Admission GCS score of 7. **a** Initial CT scan 2 h after injury shows diffuse bilateral tSAH localized in the sulci and on the left Sylvian fissure. **b** CT scan 24 h later shows progressive right frontotemporal damage with predominant hypodense anterior edema and a posterior parenchymal clot. (From [12])

15.4
Future Directions

The introduced guidelines for head injury management [9, 27, 44, 59] have attempted to standardize the management of neurotrauma patients, regardless of their being located in a hospital with or without a neurosurgical unit. Unfortunately, the application of guidelines is far from being achieved owing to obvious logistic or cultural difficulties and the unspoken triage criterion reported.

Usually, the beds of a NH represent a small percentage of the beds in a specific geographical area. Thus, the application of the guidelines in an entire area combined with transmission of images from the GH to the NH with the adoption of TR could allow a better selection of patients for referral for neurosurgery for a more rational use of resources.

An area protocol should be developed following meetings of all physicians involved in the treatment of brain injury, including neurosurgeons, intensivists, emergency physicians, pediatricians, neurologists, and general surgeons. In these meetings, the health-care organizations define the best management achievable with the application of the guidelines related to the available logistic, medical, and economical resources.

The senior author of this chapter in 2002 reported an example of regional guidelines adopted since 1998 [51], with the demonstration of how it is feasible to coordinate in an entire area the treatment of head-injured patients with a network of connected hospitals.

In Table 15.4 are summarized the guidelines reported in Servadei et al. [51], integrated with more recent observations about the high risk of progression of IPHs and tSAH. In Table 15.5 is reported the communication form adopted between a GH and a NH.

With the development of communication technologies, it is possible to organize a "hub and spoke" system where the high complexity of assistance is concentrated in centers of excellence (hub), supported by a network of services (spoke) responsible for the selection of patients and sending them to reference centers when a particular gravity is exceeded.

Table 15.4 The regional guidelines of Romagna [51] modified with respect to the presence of traumatic subarachnoid hemorrhage (*tSAH*) and/or intraparenchymal contusions and hematomas (*IPHs*) larger than 5 cm³ in the group of comatose patients

Patients with clinical deterioration and/or open head injury	Hemodynamically stabilized Transferred from the scene of injury directly to a NH	Action
All other comatose patients	Nearest GH Hemodynamically stabilized CT scan TR	DI I: sent to GH ICUs DI II: if no NH beds are available then sent to GH ICUs; CT within 12 h after injury DI II with tSAH and/or IPHs >5 cm³ sent directly to a NH DI III, IV: sent very often without transfer of images and ICU beds are released for these patients by transferring subacute patients elsewhere
Noncomatose patients	CT scan—TR	The referral is discussed case by case
Mild (GCS 14–15)		Italian national guidelines for adults (the study group)

TR teleradiology

Table 15.5 As stated in the guidelines of Romagna, the GH sends to the NH the neurodiagnostic study with TR and a fax with information about the action in the emergency room related to the patient, the trauma scores, the clinical status, and the presence of risk factors

Action in emergency room	Transit
	Admitted for worsening
	Admitted for miscellaneous reasons
	Death
	Transferred
Trauma score	GCS
	Revised trauma score (Champion)
Risk factors	Anticoagulation/antiplatelet therapy
	Drug abuse
	Alcohol abuse
	Previous neurosurgery
	Elderly
	Disability
	Epilepsy
Pupil diameter	
Breathing	Spontaneous
	Intubation
	Ventilation
	Sedation
Impact site	Frontal
	Temporal
	Parietal
	Occipital
Associated lesions	Abdomen
	Face
	Limbs
	Spine
	Thorax
Hemodynamics	Heart frequency
	Systolic pressure

The application of the hub and spoke model has three key objectives:

1. Ensure that individual neurosurgical centers can deal with a volume of activity enough to acquire and maintain clinical competence and operational efficiency.
2. Create channels of continuous communication between the referral hub and the spokes, in order to guarantee continuous availability and collaboration.
3. Encourage the development of systematic activities of clinical audit within and among centers and develop knowledge of "the area treatment" including common follow-ups.

Summary

The following are the important points discussed in the chapter:

- TR experiences from workstation to wireless technology
- Discrepancies from an "ideal world" of guidelines and a "real world" of medical practice
- The real predictive value of GCS admission for the outcome of the brain-injured patient
- Differences regarding the outcome of TBI patients treated with or without neurosurgical facilities
- How to detect the CT evolution before the neurologic change
- Application of guidelines with area protocol and "hub and spoke" systems

References

1. Armin SS, Colohan AR, Zhang JH (2006) Traumatic subarachnoid hemorrhage: our current understanding and its evolution over the past half century. Neurol Res 28(4):445–452
2. Ashkenazi I, Haspel J, Alfici R, Kessel B, Khashan T, Oren M (2007) Effect of teleradiology upon pattern of transfer of head injured patients from a rural general hospital to a neurosurgical referral centre. Emerg Med J 24(8):550–552
3. Balestreri M, Czosnyka M, Chatfield DA et al (2004) Predictive value of Glasgow Coma Scale after brain trauma: change in trend over the past ten years. J Neurol Neurosurg Psychiatry 75:161–162
4. Beaumont A, Gennarelli T (2006) CT prediction of contusion evolution after closed head injury: the role of pericontusional edema. Acta Neurochir Suppl 96:30–32
5. Brown CVR, Zada G, Salim A et al (2007) Indications for routine repeat head computed tomography (CT) stratified by severity of traumatic brain injury. J Trauma 62:1339–1345
6. Bruder N (2007) Transfer of emergency neurosurgical patients: when and how? Ann Fr Anesth Reanim 26(10):873–877

7. Bullock R, Chesnut RM, Clifton G et al (1996) Guidelines for the management of severe head injury. J Neurotrauma 11:639–734

8. Bullock RM, Zauner A, Woodward JJ et al (1998) Factors affecting excitatory amino acid release following severe human head injury. J Neurosurg 89:507–518

9. Bullock R, Chesnut R, Ghajar J et al (2006) Guidelines for the surgical management of traumatic brain injury. Neurosurgery 58(3 Suppl):S2-47-S2-55

10. Champion HR, Sacco WJ, Copes WS, Gann DS, Gennarelli TA, Flanagan ME (1989) A revision of the trauma score. J Trauma 29(5):623–629

11. Chang EF, Meeker M, Holland MC (2006) Acute traumatic intraparenchymal hemorrhage: risk factors for progression in the early post-injury period. Neurosurgery 58(4):647–656; discussion 647–656

12. Chieregato A, Fainardi E, Morselli-Labate AM et al (2005) Factors associated with neurological outcome and lesion progression in traumatic subarachnoid hemorrhage patients. Neurosurgery 56(4):671–680; discussion 671–680

13. Daucourt V, Sicotte C, Pelletier-Fleuri N, Petitjean ME, Chateil JF, Michel P (2006) Cost-minimization analysis of a wide-area teleradiology network in a French region. Int J Qual Health Care 18(4):287–293

14. Durham SR, Liu KC, Selden NR (2006) Utility of serial computed tomography imaging in pediatric patients with head trauma. J Neurosurg 105(5 Suppl):365–369

15. Fainardi E, Chieregato A, Antonelli V, Fagioli L, Servadei F (2004) Time course of CT evolution in traumatic subarachnoid haemorrhage: a study of 141 patients. Acta Neurochir (Wien) 146(3):257–263; discussion 263

16. Farin A, Deutsch R, Biegon A, Marshall LF (2003) Sex-related differences in patients with severe head injury: greater susceptibility to brain swelling in female patients 50 years of age and younger. J Neurosurg 98:32–69

17. Fins JJ (2003) Constructing an ethical stereotaxy for severe brain injury: balancing risks, benefits and access. Nat Rev 4:323–327

18. Goh KY, Lam CK, Poon WS (1997) The impact of teleradiology on the interhospital transfer of neurosurgical patients. Br J Neurosurg 11:52–56

19. Hukkelhoven CW, Steyerberg EW, Rampen AJ et al (2003) Patient age and outcome following severe traumatic brain injury: an analysis of 5600 patients. J Neurosurg 99:666–673

20. Kaups KL, Davis JW, Parks SN (2004) Routinely repeated computed tomography after blunt head trauma: does it benefit patients? J Trauma 56:475–481

21. Kim DK, Yoo SK, Kim SH (2005) Instant wireless transmission of radiological images using a personal digital assistant phone for emergency teleconsultation. J Telemed Telecare 11(Suppl 2):S58–S61

22. Kim DK, Yoo SK, Park JJ, Kim SH (2007) PDA-phone-based instant transmission of radiological images over a CDMA network by combining the PACS screen with a Bluetooth-interfaced local wireless link. J Digit Imaging 20(2):131–139

23. Kondo Y (2002) Medical image transfer for emergency care utilizing Internet and mobile phone. Nippon Hoshasen Gijutsu Gakkai Zasshi 58(10):1393–1401

24. Lehoux P, Sicotte C, Denis JL, Berg M, Lacroix A (2002) The theory of use behind telemedicine: how compatible with physicians' clinical routines? Soc Sci Med 54:889–904

25. Lobato RD, Gomez PA, Alday R et al (1997) Sequential computerized tomography changes and related final outcome in severe head injury patients. Acta Neurochir (Wien) 139:385–391

26. Lobato RD, Alen JF, Perez-Nuñez A et al (2005) Value of serial CT scanning and intracranial pressure monitoring for detecting new intracranial mass effect in severe head injury patients showing lesions type I-II in the initial CT scan. Neurocirugia (Astur) 16(3):217–234

27. Maas AJR, Dearden M, Teasdale GM et al (1997) EBIC-guidelines for management of severe head injury in adults. Acta Neurochir (Wien) 139:286–294

28. MacFarlane A, Harrison R, Wallace P (2002) The benefits of a qualitative approach to telemedicine research. J Telemed Telecare 8(Suppl 2):56–57

29. Marshall LF, Marshall SB, Klauber MR et al (1992) The diagnosis of head injury requires a classification based on computed axial tomography. J Neurotrauma 9(Suppl 1): S287–S292

30. McIntosh TL (1993) Novel pharmacological therapies in the treatment of experimental traumatic brain injury. J Neurotrauma 10:215–259

31. Morris K (1993) Assessment and communication of conscious level: an audit of neurosurgical referrals. Injury 24:369–372

32. Mun SK, Turner JW (1999) Telemedicine: emerging e-medicine. Annu Rev Biomed Eng 01:589–610

33. Munro PT, Smith RD, Parke TR (2002) Effect of patients' age on management of acute intracranial haematoma: prospective national study. BMJ 325:1001

34. Nathens AB, Maier RV, Copass MK, Jurkovich GJ (2001) Payer status: the unspoken triage criterion. J Trauma 50:776–783

35. National Collaborating Centre for Acute Care (2003) Head injury: triage, assessment, investigation and early management of head injury in infants, children and adults. National Health Service, National Institute for Clinical Excellence, London, p 74

36. Ng WH, Wang E, Ng I (2007) Multimedia messaging service teleradiology in the provision of emergency neurosurgery services. Surg Neurol 67(4):338–341

37. Oertel M, Kelly DF, McArthur D et al (2002) Progressive hemorrhage after head trauma: predictors and consequences of the evolving injury. J Neurosurg 96(1):109–116

38. Papo I, Caruselli G, Luongo A, Scarpelli M, Pasquini U (1980) Traumatic cerebral mass lesions: correlations between clinical, intracranial pressure, and computer tomographic data. Neurosurgery 7:337–346

39. Patel NY, Hoyt DB, Nakaji P et al (2000) Traumatic brain injury: patterns of failure of nonoperative management. J Trauma 48:367–374

40. Patel HC, Bouamra O, Woodford M et al (2005) Trends in head injury outcome from 1989 to 2003 and the effect of neurosurgical care: an observational study. Lancet 366: 1538–1544

41. Pelletier-Fleury N, Fargeon V, Lanoe JL, Fardeau M (1997) Transaction costs economics as a conceptual framework for the analysis of barriers to the diffusion of telemedicine. Health Policy 42:1–14

42. Piek J, Hebecker R, Schütze M, Sola S, Mann S, Buchholz K (2006) Image transfer by mobile phones in neurosurgery. Zentralbl Neurochir 67(4):193–196

43. Poca MA, Sahuquillo J, Domenech P et al (2004) Use of teleradiology in the evaluation and management of head-injured patients. Results of a pilot study of a link between a district general hospital and a neurosurgical referral center. Neurocirugia (Astur) 15(1):17–35

44. Procaccio F, Stocchetti N, Citerio G et al (2000) Guidelines for the treatment of adults with severe head trauma. J Neurosurg Sci 44:1–10

45. Randles TJ, Thachenkary CS (2002) Toward an understanding of diagnostic teleconsultations and their impact on diagnostic confidence. Telemed J E Health 8:377–385

46. Schuhmann MU, Rickels E, Rosahl SK, Schneekloth CG, Samii M (2001) Acute care in neurosurgery: quantity, quality, and challenges J Neurol Neurosurg Psychiatry 71: 182–187

47. Scottish Intercollegiate Guidelines Network (2000) Early management of patients with a head injury. Edinburgh: SIGN, Publication ISBN 1899893 27 X 46:36

48. Servadei F, Nanni A, Nasi MT et al (1995) Evolving brain lesions in the first 12 hours after head injury: analysis of 37 comatose patients. Neurosurgery 37(5):899–906; discussion 906–907

49. Servadei F, Murray GD, Penny K et al (2000) The value of the 'worst' computed tomographic scan in clinical studies of moderate and severe head injury. European Brain Injury Consortium. Neurosurgery 46:70–75

50. Servadei F, Nasi MT, Giuliani G et al (2000) CT prognostic factors in acute subdural haematomas: the value of the "worst" CT scan. Br J Neurosurg 14(26):110–111

51. Servadei F, Antonelli V, Mastrilli A, Cultrera F, Giuffrida M, Staffa G (2002) Integration of image transmission into a protocol for head injury management: a preliminary report. Br J Neurosurg 16(1):36–42

52. Servadei F, Murray GD, Teasdale GM et al (2002) Traumatic subarachnoid hemorrhage: demographic and clinical study of 750 patients from the European brain injury consortium survey of head injuries. Neurosurgery 50(2):261–267; discussion 267–269

53. Servadei F, Compagnone C, Sahuquillo J (2007) The role of surgery in traumatic brain injury. Curr Opin Crit Care 13:163–168

54. Shigemori M, Tokutomi T, Hirohata M, Maruiwa H, Kaku N, Kuramoto S (1990) Clinical significance of traumatic subarachnoid hemorrhage. Neurol Med Chir 30:396–400

55. Sicotte C, Lehoux P (2003) Teleconsultation: rejected and emerging uses. Methods Infect Med 42:451–457

56. Sifri ZC, Livingston DH, Lavery RF et al (2004) Value of repeat cranial computed axial tomography scanning in patients with minimal head injury. Am J Surg 187:338–342

57. Tagliaferri F, Compagnone C, Korsic M, Servadei F, Kraus J (2006) A systematic review of brain injury epidemiology in Europe. Acta Neurochir (Wien) 148:255–268

58. Tasker RC, Morris KP, Forsyth RJ, Hawley CA, Parslow RC on behalf of the UK Paediatric Brain Injury Study Group and the Paediatric Intensive Care Society Study Group (2006) Severe head injury in children: emergency access to neurosurgery in the United Kingdom. Emerg Med J 23:519–522

59. The Study Group on Head Injury of the Italian Society for Neurosurgery (1996) Guidelines for minor head injured patients' management in adult age. J Neurol Sci 40:11–15

60. Valadka AB (2006) Brain injury management: quo vadis? Clin Neurosurg 53:295–299

61. Velmahos GC, Gervasini A, Petrovick L et al (2006) Routine repeat head CT for minimal head injury is unnecessary. J Trauma 60:494–501

62. Visca A, Faccani G, Massaro F et al (2006) Clinical and neuroimaging features of severely brain-injured patients treated in a neurosurgical unit compared with patients treated in peripheral non-neurosurgical hospitals. Br J Neurosurg 20(2):82–86

63. Walters KA (1993) Telephoned head injury referrals: the need to improve the quality of information provided. Arch Emerg Med 10:29–34

64. Wang MC, Linnau KF, Tirschwell DL, Hollingsworth W (2006) Utility of repeat head computed tomography after blunt head trauma: a systematic review. J Trauma 61:226–233

65. Wong H, Poon W, Jacobs P et al (2006) The comparative impact of video consultation on emergency neurosurgical referrals. Neurosurgery 59:607–613

66. Yaghmai V, Salehi SA, Kuppuswami S, Berlin JW (2004) Rapid wireless transmission of head CT images to a personal digital assistant for remote consultation. Acad Radiol 11(11):1291–1293

67. Yamada M, Watarai H, Andou T, Sakai N (2003) Emergency image transfer system through a mobile telephone in Japan: technical note. Neurosurgery 52(4):986–988; discussion 988–990

68. Yamamoto LG (1995) Using JPEG image compression to facilitate telemedicine. Am J Emerg Med 13:55–57

69. Yamamoto LG (1995) Wireless teleradiology and fax using cellular phones and notebook PCs for instant access to consultants. Am J Emerg Med 13:184–187

70. Yamamoto LG, Suh PJ (1996) Accessing and using the Internet's world wide web for emergency physicians. Am J Emerg Med 14:302–308

71. Yamamoto LG, Williams DR (2000) A demonstration of instant pocket wireless CT teleradiology to facilitate stat neurosurgical consultation and future telemedicine implications. Am J Emerg Med 18:423–426

72. Yamamoto LG, Elliott P, Herman MI, Abramo TJ (1996) Telemedicine using the internet. Am J Emerg Med 14:416–420

73. Zulu BMW, Mulaudzi TV, Madiba TE, Muckart DJJ (2007) Outcome of head injuries in general surgical units with an off-site neurosurgical service. Injury 38:576–583

16

Impact of Teleradiology in Clinical Practice: A Malaysian Perspective

B. J. J. Abdullah

Abstract Malaysia's National Telehealth Policy project has been undertaken in order to meet the increasing demand and expectations of the population, rising health-care costs, changing demography, changing disease patterns as well as limited resources, and the persistent differentials in health status between urban and rural populations. Four main projects have been identified to promote and maintain the wellness of Malaysians and to provide greater access to health-care information for improved personal health management: the Lifetime Health Plan, Mass Customized Personal Health Information & Education, continuous medical education, and teleconsultation.

16.1
Introduction

Until recently, the need to take a patient's history and perform a physical examination, apply complex techniques or procedures, and share information quickly made medicine very much a local affair. Even though there were patients who chose to travel for care, making pilgrimages to academic Meccas for sophisticated surgery, for example, they were exceptions [24]. This localization was largely a product of medicine's physicality as well as the strong emphasis on patient–physician relationships. In most instances, data gathering required face-to-face discussions with patients and sifting through paper files and records.

However, as health care becomes digitized, many activities, ranging from diagnostic imaging to the manipulation of laparoscopic instruments, are increasingly being rendered borderless. Telemedicine was introduced in the early 1960s by scientists from NASA to monitor the physiological parameters of astronauts. Teleradiology, which is the most mature and rapidly evolving branch of telemedicine, refers to the use of computers and telecommunication networks to transmit diagnostic images acquired at one location to another for primary review and interpretation as well as specialist consultation. In addition, teleradiology requires more data capacity than other telemedicine applications. Thus, telemedicine may have a large impact on teleradiology and vice versa.

Rapid advances in telecommunications and computers have overcome many of the initial problems, and the rising cost of health care is driving the need for establishing a cost-effective and efficient communication system. Teleradiology is seen as a vehicle for maintaining quality while containing cost in a competitive marketplace where the role of private health-care providers in the overall health system is increasing. There is still controversy regarding the exact role of teleradiology, with proponents and opponents on either side. Most of these focus on the issues of economics, market share, and quality of service.

The benefits accrued to teleradiology include more timely interpretation of radiological images and greater access to secondary consultations, in addition to improved continuing medical education, the ultimate objective of which is to significantly improve patient care. With the medical tourism market estimated to grow by US $2.2 billion with a corresponding increase of US $60 billion in the health-care market [5], teleradiology will also feature prominently. Medical tourism is a rapidly growing industry even in the so-called developing countries, with countries like Mexico, Brazil, Costa Rica, Dominican Republic, Lithuania, Hungary, Israel, Jordan, South Africa, India, Malaysia, Thailand, and the Philippines actively promoting it [10].

Nevertheless, the current objectives of teleradiology revolve around the ultimate role of making a primary diagnosis from transmitted images without review of the original images, thus providing consultative and interpretative radiological services. Teleradiology plays important roles in the following areas:

- In remote areas
- In medical facilities without on-site radiological support
- In emergent and nonemergent clinical care areas
- In on-call situations
- In subspecialty areas
- Continuous medical education (CME) for practicing radiologists
- For efficiency and quality improvement
- Sending interpreted images to the referring doctors
- For direct supervision of off-site imaging studies
- For remote treatment using robotic surgery [9]

Malaysia has a population of 27.17 million, of which 38% reside in rural areas [8]. The Malaysian government's major priority has been the enhancement of health of "disadvantaged" rural communities, particularly the rural poor, women, infants, children, and the disabled, as well as enhancement of the quality of services being provided by the general and district hospitals. The Ministry of Health is the main health-care provider, with general practitioners and the private health-care facilities playing a complementary role. Improvement in health status of the rural population using universal health status indicators has been remarkable. However, as a result of increasing demand and expectations of the population, rising health-care costs, changing demography, changing disease patterns as well as limited resources, and the persistent differentials in health status between urban and rural populations, Malaysia's National Telehealth Policy [16] project is seen as a means of achieving improved quality of health. It has a clear, strategic, and long-term plan and policies implemented for e-health [13]. As a consequence, it is envisioned that the health services would be more integrated, coordinated, cost-effective, and available to those in need, with the maximum use of existing resources and modern technology. In addition, the health services should be available for both management of wellness and illnesses [23].

16.2
History of Teleradiology in Malaysia

As a result of constraints on the number and expertise of neurosurgeons in Malaysia in the 1990s, an international teleconsultation/teleradiology project was conducted between the Department of Neurosurgery of Hokkaido University School of Medicine, Japan, and the Division of Neurosurgery of Universiti Kebangsaan Malaysia, Malaysia, beginning in March 1995. During this period, neurosurgeons from both places discussed several cases of carotid cavernous fistula (CCF), cerebral arteriovenous malformation (AVM), and large vertebral artery aneurysm, which need endovascular treatment, by mailing radiological data and sending faxes. Japanese physicians visited Malaysia again and treated several patients with CCF and AVM by using endovascular surgical techniques. The results were satisfactory, as two patients with CCF and aneurysm completely recovered and partial embolization of the deep-seated AVM was achieved in one patient. The cost performance was almost equal to that of the conventional mailing system. The most remarkable advantage of this new system is the high quality of transferred images (transmission of one image took approximately 20 s), the cost and time performance, and the security of the medical information [6].

Two connections were established between Selayang Hospital and Kuala Lumpur Hospital (KLH). The first connection was established between the Emergency Department of Selayang Hospital and the call center of KLH, primarily for neurosurgical referral. The second connection was established between the diagnostic imaging departments of both hospitals [7].

In November 1995, the Malaysian government formally announced the setting up of a specialized designated zone called the "multimedia super corridor," designed to leapfrog Malaysia into the information and knowledge age. It includes an area of approximately $15 \times 50\,km^2$, which stretches from the Petronas Twin Towers to Kuala Lumpur International Airport and also includes the towns of Putrajaya and Cyberjaya, including the entire Klang Valley. This was Malaysia's most exciting initiative for the global information and communication technology (ICT) industry.

Many innovative flagship applications were formulated and implemented in MSC Malaysia to accelerate its growth. Those were focused on the development of smart schools, telehealth, e-business, smart-card technology, electronic government, and technopreneurship. The latest flagship application is the Creative Multimedia cluster, which aims to catalyze the development of the Malaysian creative content industry in Malaysia, engaging the participation of global producers. Furthermore, Cyberjaya is finding its niche as a regional outsourcing and shared services haven for international companies.

The objectives of the telehealth initiative of the MSC initiatives are to promote and maintain the wellness of Malaysians and to provide greater access to health-care information for improved personal health management. Four main projects have been identified. First is the Lifetime Health Plan (LHP), which generates focused, proactive personal health maintenance and enhances individuals' quality of life. Currently, the services are available online at the main hospitals and 24 health clinics. Patient records (LHP) will be available on demand by any authorized caregiver, from any location, any time of the day, and this will go beyond videoconferencing, as it will integrate the transmission of digitized patient records, including diagnostic images in real time or in store-and-forward mode. It is hoped that this will help to improve the equity of access to quality care, especially to underserved areas, and realize the goal of care closer to the patient's home.

Second is the Mass Customized Personal Health Information & Education (MCPHIE), which empowers the public with education and wellness information for personalized health maintenance. Currently, there are 1,298 Web pages of accredited health content. Third is the CME, which provides the best available medical knowledge to health-care professionals on a timely basis. Currently, live registration can be done at the online portal site. Finally, the fourth project is teleconsultation, which provides electronic peer information sharing capabilities for the development of excellence in patient diagnosis. More than 1,000 referrals have been carried out for live cases (e.g., teleradiology, teledermatology, and telecardiology) [20].

The teleconsultation application's primary objective is to provide specialist care to remote health clinics and health centers where there is a lack of specialists. This is done by connecting a combination of health-care providers and patients in a multipoint manner (teleconsultation links) to share opinions, provide support, and deliver care to patients at home or close to their homes. On January 20, 2000, a telemedicine signing ceremony between MSC Malaysia and the Ministry of Health was witnessed by the then Health Minister Dato' Chua Jui Meng.

In January 2000, WorldCare (an affiliate of WorldCare Limited) was awarded the MSC Teleconsultation Flagship Application by the Malaysian Government to manage and operate it from April 2000 to October 2002 under an RM 20 million allocation. The service was continued until July 2003, when it was temporarily disrupted. This pilot project was scheduled to link 41 government health-care centers and hospitals, located strategically throughout Malaysia, into an integrated teleconsultation network. The initial focus of this new service was supposed to include cardiovascular, cancer antenatal/perinatal, trauma, and emergency medical teleconsultation. The software, hardware, installation, technical support, operational training, and maintenance to facilitate consultation between patients and physicians via linked medical instruments and imaging systems were provided by WorldCare Health (Malaysia). (WCHM).

This project was unique in being one of the world's first nationally established telemedicine networks. In a unique public–private partnership, the Malaysian government permitted the use of the network to meet the needs of private physicians and patients. With use of its FDA-approved OpenMed™ platform, designed for WorldCare's Global Telemedicine Network, technologies will empower the Malaysian network, deploying an intelligent, multimodality, multispecialty, clinical management platform for the creation, management, referral, transmission, storage, and display of a multimedia computerized patient record. WCHM was selected on a competitive basis to lead this project and, will, under the guidance of the Malaysian Ministry of Health, be solely responsible for implementing the teleconsultation application program structured under the auspices of Malaysia's new MSC initiative. It became fully operational in Sabah in March 2002. In Sabah, it links four district hospitals, i.e., Semporna, Beluran, Ranau, and Kudat, to the hub at Queen Elizabeth Hospital (QEH). The software is a Windows-based system designed and developed by WCHM, which was also providing the technical maintenance and training needs. All these sites are connected using integrated services digital network (ISDN) lines. In Sabah, a teleradiology service is available 24 h a day to the four district hospitals. It is not designed to be a film reporting system but more for consultation on problem and difficult cases. The district medical officers are encouraged to refer radiographs for radiologists' opinion so as to assist them in managing the patients.

In the first 5 months (March–July 2002) of the service, a total of 90 cases were referred for radiological opinion. The radiographs referred for opinion included chest radiographs, which formed the majority (about 70%); abdominal radiographs; skeletal radiographs; and a few intravenous urograms. These cases were from a variety of medical disciplines (medicine, surgery, orthopedic surgery, and pediatrics). There were also five referrals from QEH to KLH for neurosurgical opinion and one each for urology and hepatobiliary surgical opinion, based on computed tomography scans performed at QEH. On average, the four district hospitals will get a reply in 6 h, whereas for the other district hospitals it will take an average of 2 weeks to do so using the conventional method of sending the radiograph through the ambulance service (C.K. Lim, consultant radiologist, Sabah, personal communication).

In Malaysia, there was a proliferation of vendors who have been marketing their teleradiology systems but have not informed the users about their true capabilities. The end users are, however, lost as to the requirements of a teleradiology system. It is essential that any teleradiology system provides images of sufficient quality, without significant loss of spatial or contrast resolution from image acquisition through transmission to final image display. For transmission of images for display only, the image quality should be sufficient to satisfy the needs of the clinical scenario. As all these concerns of the radiological community regarding the safety of teleradiology are being promoted and used, the College of Radiology, Academy of Medicine, Malaysia (http://www.radiologymalaysia.org), decided to formulate guidelines on the use of teleradiology. These guidelines were adapted from the guidelines issued by the American College of Radiology on Standards on Teleradiology as well as the Royal College of Radiologists, UK, and hoped to define the objectives of a teleradiology system; minimum requirements of the hardware and software; training; qualifications of personnel, including licensing, credentialing, and liability; network and communication requirements; quality control; and the need for quality improvement for teleradiology.

In the wider community, further projects are also being explored. One such project is the development of teleradiology software (RadArt) involving researchers at Universiti Putra Malaysia, Universiti Sains Malaysia, Universiti Teknologi Mara, and the Malaysian Institute of Nuclear Technology and Research [21]. Complete and powerful teleradiology software, namely, RadArt, which a cost-effective solution for performing real-time interactive remote expert consultation for radiograph procedures, has been developed at the Universiti Teknologi Malaysia (UTM). It is a joint research and development project between the Faculty of Computer Science and Information Technology of UTM and Syarikat Datarunding. The project was made possible with the assistance from various organizations, including the Ministry of Science, Technology, and Environment through its Malaysian Teaching Company Scheme grant, Syarikat Telekom Malaysia by providing an ISDN line, and the Radiology Department of Hospital

University Sains Malaysia by providing expert opinion. Other notable developments have been research initiatives involving the use of different compression algorithms [19].

Malaysia's Teleconsultation Network was reactivated in June 2005 with an allocation of RM 6.3 million for maintenance, upgrading of equipment, and telecommunications services. In the most recent government initiative in May 2007, 38 hospitals across the country were linked by digitized telecommunications under an RM 27 million program. This follows on from a successful pilot project using radiographs, echocardiograms, laboratory results, and coronary arteriograms to determine the health of patients. For a start, teleconsultation, one of the major applications of telemedicine, is being used for five disciplines: radiology, cardiology, dermatology, accident and traumatology, and neurosurgery. Put in place by WCHM, it also allows for peer-to-peer transmission of film-based radiological images as well as scanned paper documents, voice annotations, digital images, and echocardiogram scans. Responses can be expected between 30 min and 24 h after a request has been made. The services can be transmitted over ordinary telephone lines. If the program proves to be a success without hitches, it will be extended to other hospitals nationwide [4].

Since its inception, MSC Malaysia has grown into a thriving dynamic ICT hub, hosting more than 900 multinational and foreign-owned and home-grown Malaysian companies focused on multimedia and communications products, solutions, services, and research and development. With this unique corridor, Malaysia continues to attract leading ICT companies from around the world to locate their industries in MSC Malaysia and undertake research, develop new products and technologies, and export from this base. MSC Malaysia is also an ideal growth environment for Malaysian ICT small and medium-sized enterprises to transform themselves into world-class companies. Furthermore, MSC Malaysia welcomes countries to use its highly advanced infrastructural facilities as a global test bed for ICT applications and a hub for their regional operations in Asia [14].

16.3
Lessons Learned and Future Challenges

Skyrocketing health-care costs are increasingly seen as unsustainable drains on public coffers, corporate profits, and household savings. Concern about these costs has led to wide-ranging cost-cutting efforts, often accompanied by attempts to improve quality and safety. Also, many hospitals now purchase interpretation services from outside companies, whose interpreters often speak a range of languages that individual hospitals cannot match. Outsourcing could also provide patients with access to specialized care that would otherwise be unavailable. In other areas of the economy, a similar search for cost savings and value has created a powerful impetus for outsourcing [24]. With the increased role of globalization and barriers being brought down, albeit slowly, outsourcing usually triumphs. In addition, partners retire, radiologists become sick or injured, everyone in health care needs a vacation, and the demand for imaging services seems to grow exponentially every year. The new mantra of doing more with less under these circumstances eventually becomes a zero-sum game and threatens professional burnout to those left to pick up the extra work.

The offshore interpretation of radiologic studies is the proof that technology and the political and economic climate will now permit the outsourcing of medical care, a trend with profound implications for health-care policy and practice. Diagnostic imaging reading service groups have grown and evolved over the past decade to seamlessly step in and remotely provide the expertise needed to reduce an imaging practice's workload. Teleradiology services are now available for every imaging subspecialty and perform preliminary as well as final reads 24 h a day, 7 days a week, 365 days a year. These providers actively work to partner with a practice, taking on the roll of clinical colleagues for a group's customers and referring clinicians.

In brief, there are several lessons that can be learned from the experiences of the implementation of teleradiology programs in Malaysia. Firstly, it requires a realistic assessment, particularly a very clear policy, committed leadership, an implementation program, and the right technology frameworks recognizing that the technology is an enabler and not the solution. Teleradiology also requires a pragmatic approach, taking into consideration the locality environments, capabilities, and requirements, among others. Even though similar initiatives have succeeded elsewhere, they may not succeed simply because the technology is available, i.e., what is technologically possible may not be organizationally or socially or politically possible. The financial resources to continuously upgrade the hardware and software are another vital component to the success of this program. Finally, the implementation of a successful national telemedicine/teleradiology program practically requires marketing expertise to better promote awareness, encouragement, and dissemination of information on the benefits that can be reaped by the citizens and other stakeholders.

Instead of patient data being archived or managed by hospitals or national organizations, there is a growing trend for individuals to record their medical information on Web sites [17] or devices that the attending physician then accesses to make treatment decisions. One such device is the Medstick [5], a portable device that enables you to have all relevant medical data with you

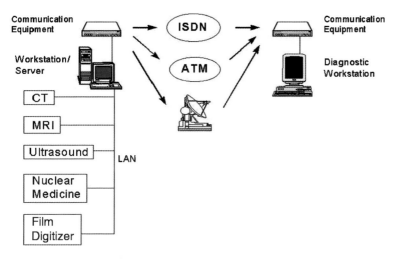

Fig. 16.1. The impact of teleradiology in clinical practice—a Malaysian perspective [2]

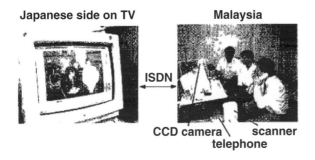

Fig. 16.2. Television conference [6]

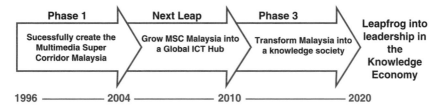

Fig. 16.3. The MSC Malaysia vision from 1996 to 2020 [14]

Integrated Telehealth Chart

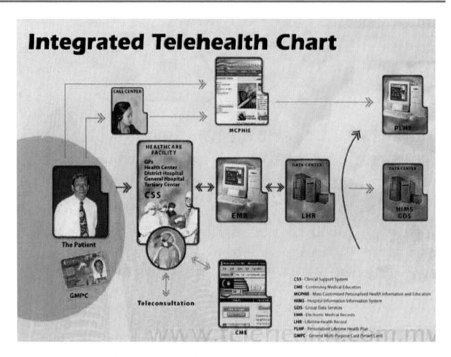

Fig. 16.4. Integrated telehealth chart [13]

wherever you go, including an emergency field, imaging studies, and a medical database. Then there are those that allow you to have the information on your palmtop [11]. Teleradiology is not far behind. Continuing miniaturization and standardization of microchip technology in personal digital assistants (PDAs) with increased speeds and data storage, screens with better color depth, display quality, dedicated graphics acceleration hardware, and standardization of operating software now make it possible for interactive image manipulation and analysis. The costs have also decreased significantly. PDAs are capable of serving as a powerful platform for mobile image review and management. As high-speed wireless networks become ubiquitous, personal handheld devices will become an important platform for image review and reporting in the radiology department workflow and will enhance communication with referring clinicians. The development of a PDA-based, DICOM-compatible teleradiology system that is capable of vendor-independent seamless integration with a picture archiving and communication system is inevitable [22].

Thus, instead of relying on a national and complicated centralized system, the personal medical database and personal devices are going to be the new face of telehealth and teleradiology [3, 18].

16.4
Conclusion

People, organizations, and countries will find a niche where they are most competitive. No specialty will be spared, from the radiologists to cardiologists to surgeons to radiation oncologists, etc. For some countries, it will be good-quality health care at low cost; for others, it will be the highest-quality health care at a higher cost; and for those in places like Bangkok, Dubai, and Buenos Aires, it will be a geographical advantage. What is happening in the globalization of trade in health is individual countries with certain strategic competitive advantages, be they quality, cost, or geographical convenience, are exploiting them to the fullest. Health tourism centers/clinics are actively seeking First World "customers" by increasingly pursuing and adopting American and other international best practices to maintain the quality of services [1, 15].

If medical information, images, and diagnosis become mere "commodities" that can be sought, bought, traded, and sold over the Internet, then the only real option left for the medical specialists is to add value [12] by synthesizing all the disparate pieces of information in the context of each individual patient locally, to optimize the selection of treatment and therefore outcomes. Additionally, the physician must continue to be protective in guiding and showing care for the patient [1].

Summary

- Teleradiology, which is the most mature and rapidly evolving branch of telemedicine, uses computers and telecommunication networks to transmit diagnostic images and data from one location to another for primary review and interpretation as well as specialist consultation.
- Malaysia's National Telehealth Policy [16] project has been undertaken in order to meet the increasing demand and expectations of the population, rising health-care costs, changing demography, changing disease patterns as well as limited resources, and the persistent differentials in health status between urban and rural populations.
- In November 1995, the Malaysian government announced the setting up of a specialized designated zone called the "multimedia super corridor," Malaysia's most exciting initiative for the global ICT industry.
- Four main projects have been identified to promote and maintain the wellness of Malaysians and to provide greater access to health-care information for improved personal health management: the LHP, MCPHIE, CME, and teleconsultation.

References

1. Abdullah BJ, Ng KH (2006) The sky is falling. Biomed Eng Interv J 2(3):e29
2. Abdullah BJ, Ng KH, Pathmanathan R (1999) The impact of teleradiology in clinical practice—a Malaysian perspective. Med J Malaysia 54(2):169–174
3. Banitsas KA, Georgiadis P, Tachakra S, Cavouras D (2004) Using handheld devices for real-time wireless teleconsultation. Paper presented at the 26th Annual international conference of the IEEE EMBS, San Francisco
4. Cruez AF (2007) Medicine's here: now you can fall sick anywhere in Malaysia. New Straits Times 27 May 2007, p 26
5. EMT Alert.com (2006) Online electronic medical records storage system databases. http://www.emtalert.com/aboutus.php EMT. Last Accessed April 30, 2008
6. Houkin K, Fukuhara S, Selladurai BM et al (1999) Telemedicine in neurosurgery using international digital telephone services between Japan and Malaysia—technical note. Neurol Med Chir 39(11):773–777; discussion 7–8
7. Ministry of Health, Malaysia http://hselayang.moh.gov.my/modules/xt_conteudo/index.php?id=6. Accessed 30 April 2008
8. Department of Statistics, Govt of Malaysia (2007) Key statistics. http://www.statistics.gov.my/english/frameset_keystats.php. Accessed 30 April, 2008
9. Marescaux J, Leroy J, Rubino F et al (2002) Transcontinental robot-assisted remote telesurgery: feasibility and potential applications. Ann Surg 235(4):487–492
10. Medical tourism (2007) http://en.wikipedia.org/wiki/Health_tourism. Cited 23 April Accessed 30 April, 2008
11. Medstick: a portable personal medical database (2007) http://www.angelfire.com/journal2/medstick. Accessed 30 April 2008
12. Miles SA, Ashby MD (2002) Factors affecting leadership and human capital management. Oxford University Press, Oxford
13. Mohan J, Razali Raja Yaacob R (2004) The Malaysian Telehealth Flagship Application: a national approach to health data protection and utilisation and consumer rights. Int J Med Inform 73(3):217–227
14. MSC Malaysia (formerly known as the Multimedia Super Corridor) (2007) http://www.msc.com.my/msc/msc.asp. Accessed 30 April 2008
15. Mumbai ENB (2006) Practising medical tourism: a resounding success. http://www.expresshealthcaremgmt.com/200603/medicaltourismconf01.shtml. Accessed 30 April 2008
16. Ministry of Health, Malaysia (1999) National telehealth policy. In: Malaysia MoH (ed)
17. Raman B, Raman R, Raman L, Beaulieu CF (2004) Radiology on handheld devices: image display, manipulation, and PACS integration issues. Radiographics 24(1):299–310
18. Reponena J, Niinimäkia J, Kumpulainenb T, Ilkkoa E, Karttunena A, Jarttia P (2005) Mobile teleradiology with smartphone terminals as a part of a multimedia electronic patient record. International congress series CARS 2005. Comput Assist Radiol Surg 1281:916–921
19. Saffor A, Ramli AR, Ng KH (2001) A Comparative study of image compression between JPEG and wavelet. Malays J Comput Sci 14:39–45
20. Salleh SM (2003) The multimedia super corridor (MSC) and E-government initiatives in Malaysia. http://purple.giti.waseda.ac.jp/Bulletin/2003/2003papers/2003general_03_sohaimi.pdf. Accessed 30 April, 2008
21. Sharif R (2005) Government to launch national grid computing project. The Star. p 9

22. Solutions DD (2006) Personal medical history. http://www.biohealthmatics.com. Accessed 30 April 2008

23. Suleiman AB (2001) Telemedicine & Telehealth Networks National Networks. http://www.med.umich.edu/telemedicine/symposium/suleiman.ppt. Accessed 30 April 2008

24. Wachter RM (2006) The "dis-location" of U.S. medicine—the implications of medical outsourcing. N Engl J Med 354(7):661–665

17

Teleradiology: A Northern Finland Perspective

Jarmo Reponen

Abstract Teleradiology has been a forerunner in developing telemedicine and eHealth services in Finland. This is especially true for the Oulu University Hospital responsibility area, which is situated in the northernmost part of the country. That area covers nearly half of the Finnish territory, also including the arctic regions. Because of vast distances and a sparse population, regular teleradiology started in 1990 and has resulted in the establishment of teleradiology and televideoconferencing services, distance education, and a multimedia medical record with remote-access capabilities. Wireless technology has been a special focus area, as has the development of efficient communication between primary and secondary care. This review highlights the position of teleradiology in the spectrum of telemedicine services.

17.1
Teleradiology Background

Teleradiology is currently one of the most widely utilized telemedicine applications. The history of teleradiology in Oulu dates back to 1969, when radiological images were transmitted between Helsinki and Oulu using the broadcasting network of Finnish national television. The results of that pilot project showed that remote diagnosis was possible with great accuracy. However, the use of television broadcasting at that time was too expensive and unpractical for clinical work. That is why it was not before 1990 when modern teleradiology in our region started, using first videoconferencing using multiple lines and, since 1991, digital data connections [10].

The teleradiology development program consisted of three major areas: teleradiology for primary health care, teleradiology for secondary care (hospitals), and the development of mobile teleradiology. In the development phase, all of the projects were subjected to health technology assessment. The Finnish national criteria for technology assessment within the field of telemedicine were developed in 1996 [8] by Oulu University Hospital and the Finnish Office for Health Technology Assessment (FinOHTA).

Teleradiology serving primary health care started in 1991, using integrated services digital network lines and low-cost scanners and microcomputers. The first target was to develop the technical backbone and a business model [12]. During the last few years, the technology has seen an evolution to broadband connections and direct digital imaging and communication in medicine (DICOM) compatible interfaces between sending and receiving sites. Workflow and work practice studies have shown how technology affects cooperation between different institutions [4, 5]. The hospital network between various hospitals in northern Finland was built during 1992–1996. The network has, since that time, served for secondary opinion and emergency coverage between Oulu University Hospital and all the central, regional, and local hospitals. Assessment studies have shown that teleradiology is cost-effective and influences both patient transportation and treatment [9].

As part of the secondary opinion network, an international teleradiology network connection was established, as early as in 1993, between the university hospitals of Oulu (Finland), Reykjavik (Iceland), and Tromsoe (Norway). This was made possible by the Nordic University Network "Nordunet," which was a precursor of the public Internet. All the named centers had just purchased their first magnetic resonance imaging (MRI) scanners, and they needed secondary opinion for rare neuroradiological cases. Teleradiology provided a method to communicate with an expert from another country and to gain mutual experience faster than usual. To our knowledge, this was one of the first international teleradiology connections in the world [11, 13].

17.2
Images Are Part of a Modern Electronic Patient Record

Teleradiology alone does not sufficiently improve patient information logistics; therefore, Oulu University Hospital started a Web-based multimedia medical record project in 1995. One purpose of this development was the creation of regional eHealth services. Currently, the system, called ESKO, is used in all of the departments with currently over 300,000 registered patients. The information can be retrieved via text terminals, Web browsers, and mobile communicator devices. The patient record is a virtual record retrieved from various hospital databases, according to the users' requests. The system is technically divided into three layers: (1) user interfaces using a standard Web browser, (2) middleware taking care of the query/retrieval processes, and (3) modular databases [18].

Currently, the multimedia content of the medical record combines narrative texts, laboratory results, radiological information system information, and scanned graphics and DICOM format radiological images, such as computed tomography (CT) and computed radiology, ultrasound, and MRI scans. Together with a structured nursing care record system, there are over 3,000 professional users. With the system provided, users are able to use a familiar interface, the Web-based electronic patient record (EPR), to display almost all of the clinical data they need in the university hospital environment. Current developments include installations in three other central hospitals in Finland and secure connections to remote primary health-care centers for teleconsultations and e-referrals.

The modern medical record is a portal that can deliver information to the point of care. The integration of medical imaging should be seamless. In our hospital, the users can access all the images in DICOM archives through the EPR interface, and this approach, developed in the RUBIS project funded by the European Union, has been successful [16]. New components of the medical records can be added according to user needs and connected using standard interfaces. National and regional electronic medical guidelines are also available for the professionals through the same interface. This enforces the use of evidence-based medicine. The portal-type medical record is also a platform for mobile services for citizens and professionals. Our patients can, for example, receive health information like laboratory data via their global system for mobile communication (GSM) mobile phones, using the short message service facility.

17.3
Electronic Multimedia Communication Between Primary and Secondary Care

Today, all the primary health-care centers in northern Finland area are equipped with fully operational, paperless EPRs. This means that e-referrals and discharge letters are key tools in sharing multidisciplinary patient information between primary and secondary care. In order to be effective in a major health-care service network, e-referrals should be connected to local EPR systems and patient databases. In 1999, the first e-referral services between EPR systems at the university hospital and primary-care centers in the region were started [21]. This supplements the current network of e-consultation tools, such as teleradiology, videoconsultation services in surgery and psychiatry, and e-learning opportunities for professionals [3, 6].

There are two different ways to use our e-referral and discharge letter services: either in the form of a standardized XML message between the EPRs, or as a secure Web link. If a Web link is used, the interface gives the primary-care physician extended access to patient information in the hospital information system. If the patient has given his/her permission, the physician can read all of the multimedia information relating to a particular hospital visit. All narratives, laboratory results, and full-resolution radiological images are available online. This makes separate teleradiology connections unnecessary if only review of previous imaging studies is needed. All of the connections are protected from intruders. The primary health-care centers are connected to the university hospital over either a virtual local-area network or a virtual private network.

At present, all the 17 different university clinics provide e-referral services (emergency department; internal medicine; surgery; radiology; pediatrics; ophthalmology; neurology; neurosurgery; gynecology; radiation therapy; anesthetics; medical genetics; physical medicine/rehabilitation (physiatry); ear, nose, and throat; audiology; psychiatry; and dermatology). The target is to include all of the clinics as service providers before the end of 2004. Also all the municipalities in the responsibility area are using the services for their primary health-care centers. According to users, e-consultation is a major modification in the patient care process and has required a careful roll-out process [17].

17.4
Wireless Teleradiology

Some clinical specialties, such as neurosurgery, are dependent on image information before they can give their advice. Similarly, during on-call hours, radiology residents need to consult their seniors, who may be absent from the hospital. Our mobile teleradiology development started in 1993 with a portable wireless Nokia data phone and a laptop computer. The system showed the technical feasibility but weighed over 10 kg, so it was not taken into clinical use. In 1995, the first feasibility studies were made with a system built into a small suitcase, and, in 1997, the first smart-phone application was brought into use. Our early experiences showed that wireless devices are capable of receiving diagnostic image information [1, 14, 15].

During the years 1998–2000, the European Union provided financial support for the Mobile Medical Data (MOMEDA) project, which, according to our knowledge, produced the first pocket-sized multimedia patient record terminal for physicians. The new concept of mobile medicine means sending information to the point of expertise, or fetching information to the point of care, even outside the hospital. According to the concept, a MOMEDA server was established in the hospital intranet. In the case of consultation, the server receives the DICOM images and sends them, together with relevant narratives retrieved form the hospital EPR system, to the mobile device. The package is then forwarded to the mobile client using a GSM data pathway. Data connection is established with a secure callback method, and connections are authenticated with double-security verification. The client software is running in a Nokia communicator device, which is a smart-phone combining a pocket-sized personal digital assistant with an integrated GSM phone. The client image viewer software developed is a light-weight version of diagnostic image workstation viewer software, which is capable of full diagnostic manipulation of the data. Additional information requests can be made from the hospital EPR system, using a Web browser. Finally, a consultation phone call can be made to the hospital with a hands-free phone, while simultaneously reading the images [7].

The concept was evaluated in a real clinical setting by a team of neuroradiologists and neurosurgeons. The diagnostic quality was adequate, and user acceptance for specific emergency tasks was high. Our demonstrator showed that it is medically sensible to use pocket-sized teleradiology terminals for consultation purposes in radiology and neurosurgery. This meant that the final product was adopted for clinical use by the neurosurgeons of Oulu University Hospital in June 2000.

During the years 2002–2004, the European Union supported the Professional Mobile Data Systems (PROMODAS) project, which further developed the ideas to 2.5 generation wireless networks and platforms. The development of mobile Internet protocol networks with general packet radio system technology made it possible to stay connected with less costs than previously. New portable terminal devices with faster processors enabled a more efficient processing and display of patient information. In practice, the PROMODAS terminal replaced the earlier generation in clinical use [18].

17.5
Education and Training

As discussed before, one of the main drivers for teleradiology has been secondary opinion. This aspect has been tested, when new modalities like MRI were introduced into smaller hospitals. The statistics show that the use of teleradiology consultations then decreases in the course of time, because the local staff gain more experience. However, there are always rare cases where expert opinion is needed. Radiology reports delivered through teleradiology also supply continuous medical education to the staff of primary health centers. The introduction of picture archiving and communication systems (PACS) and filmless radiology departments has made special training for teleradiology unnecessary. Images are interpreted on computer workstations, and for radiologists there is no difference if they are reading images obtained from a CT scanner 10 m away or from a remote hospital 100 km away. There is, anyway, concern about adequate information in remote requesting. The quality of the radiologist's report is related to the clinical information he or she has received, and it is naturally easier to arrange enough information in local systems.

17.6
Current National Trends in Teleradiology

The center of excellence for telehealth, Finntelemedicum, conducted a comprehensive survey on the usage of information technology in health care in Finland, together with the Finnish National Research Centre for Welfare, in 2003 and 2005. Concerning radiology, the number of hospital districts utilizing PACS for filmless radiology increased from six of 21 to 15 of 21 between the survey years 2003 and 2005. According to the present plans, all the 21 hospital districts will be filmless before the end of 2008. This trend has had a direct influence on the teleradiology services. While 13 out of 21 hospital districts were using either traditional point-to-point teleradiology or regional image distribution in 2003, this number increased to 18 out of 21 in 2005. Some of the health-care service providers also indicated changes in technology: regional on-demand archives have taken over the role of earlier point-to-point connection, which required more labor for image transmission [2, 19].

Outsourcing of radiology services is a new phenomenon, which may become an even more important reason for teleradiology than emergency consultations or secondary opinion. The main driving factor for outsourcing is the lack of radiologists in many western European countries. Oulu University Hospital has been outsourcing the chest and bone radiographs made during off-hours in the regional emergency room. This pilot project has been running now for more than 1 year, and the first results are available. The goal was to release the burden on the staff radiologists and enable them to perform more complicated examinations. According to customer opinion, the target was achieved; there were no such rush hours at the radiology department as before. Also the emergency department received their reports in a shorter time than before [20].

17.7
Future Directions

Teleradiology services can be utilized to their full potential only if these are integrated with EPR systems. It is seen that Internet technology is a glue for system integration and gives us a useful user interface when we have to access several systems simultaneously. Development work requires continuous effort, with technical developers and users working closely together in order to find new solutions. The standardization of information contents and formats is needed for data exchange between institutions. The Finnish national project for improving health care places special emphasis on developing standards and recommendations for more secure and efficient communications. Interoperability between the various EPR systems has, since 2003, increased because of the use of a common core patient data set and a uniform coding system. A new law in Finland since July 1, 2007 makes it mandatory for all Finnish health service providers to store their electronic patient data in one national long-term archive. This capability must be achieved by 2011. After that date, all nonemergency delivery of EPR narratives, laboratory data, and images between institutions should take place via this national archive. At the moment, it is not clear if this type of connection is fast enough for emergency teleradiology. One positive influence is, however, clear: the interfaces between various hospital information and data storage systems will be standardized. The patient is the final winner when medical professionals can access information in the most practical way.

Summary

The important aspects of teleradiology discussed in this chapter are as follows:

- Development of teleradiology
- Teleradiology and multimedia medical record
- Information exchange between primary and secondary care
- Wireless teleradiology
- Teaching aspects
- Outsourcing of services
- Standardized future

Acknowledgments

The author would like to thank the European Union 4th Framework Health Telematics and 5th Framework Information Society Technology programs for supporting the MOMEDA, RUBIS, and PROMODAS projects.

References

1. Caramella D, Reponen J, Fabbrini F, Bartolozzi C (2000) Teleradiology in Europe. Eur J Radiol 33:2–7

2. Hämäläinen P, Reponen J, Winblad, (2007) eHealth of Finland. Check point 2006. STAKES reports 1/2007. STAKES, Helsinki, Finland. http://www.stakes.fi/verkkojulkaisut/raportit/R1-2007-VERKKO.pdf

3. Haukipuro K, Ohinmaa A, Winblad I, Linden T, Vuolio S (2000) The feasibility of telemedicine for orthopaedic outpatient clinics—a randomized controlled trial. J Telemed Telecare 6:193–198

4. Karasti H (1997) Using video to join analysis of work practice and system design. A study of an experimental teleradiology system and its redesign. In: Braa K, Monteiro E (eds) Proceedings of the 20th information systems research seminar in Scandinavia, "Social informatics" (IRIS'20), August 9–12, 1997. Department of Informatics, University of Oslo, pp 237–254

5. Karasti H, Reponen J, Tervonen O, Kuutti K (1998) The teleradiology system and changes in work practices. Comput Methods Programs Biomed 57(1–2):69–78

6. Mielonen ML, Ohinmaa A, Moring J, Isohanni M (1998) The use of videoconferencing for telepsychiatry in Finland. J Telemed Telecare 4:125–131

7. Niinimäki J, Holopainen A, Kerttula J, Reponen J (2001) Security development of a pocket-sized teleradiology consultation system. Medinfo 10(Pt 2):1266–1270

8. Ohinmaa A, Reponen J, Working Group (1997) A model for the assessment of telemedicine and a plan for testing of the model within five specialities. FinOHTA report 5, August 1997. http://finohta.stakes.fi/FI/julkaisut/raportit/raportti5.htm. Accessed 19 Oct 2007

9. Ohinmaa A, Nuutinen L, Reponen J (eds) (2002) Telelääketieteen arviointi Pohjois-Pohjanmaan sairaanhoitopiirissä (Assessment of telemedicine in the northern Ostrobothnia hospital district). FinOHTA report 20. http://finohta.stakes.fi/FI/julkaisut/raportit/raportti20.htm. Accessed 19 Oct 2007

10. Reponen J (2004) Radiology as a part of a comprehensive telemedicine and eHealth network in northern Finland. Int J Circumpolar Health 63(3):301–452

11. Reponen J, Palsson T, Sund T et al (1994) Nordic Teleradiology and Telemedicine Consultation Network. Proceedings of EuroPACS '94, OSIRIS Publications, Geneva

12. Reponen J, Lahde S, Tervonen O, Ilkko E, Rissanen T, Suramo I (1995) Low-cost digital teleradiology. Eur J Radiol 19(3):226–231

13. Reponen J, Palsson T, Kjartansson O et al (1995) Nordic Telemedicine Consultation Network using Internet. In: Lemke HU, Inamura K, Jaffe CC, Vannier MW (eds) Proceedings of CAR 1995. Spinger, Berlin, pp 723–728

14. Reponen J, Ilkko E, Jyrkinen L et al (1998) Digital wireless radiology consultations with a portable computer. J Telemed Telecare 4:201–205

15. Reponen J, Ilkko E, Jyrkinen L et al (2000) Initial experience with a wireless personal digital assistant as a teleradiology terminal for reporting emergency computerized tomography scans. J Telemed Telecare 6:45–49

16. Reponen J, Niinimäki J, Leinonen T, Korpelainen J, Oikarinen J, Vierimaa E (2001) Linking a web based electronic record with a DICOM PACS. In: Lemke HU et al (eds) Proceedings of CARS 2001. Elsevier, Berlin, pp 801–804

17. Reponen J, Marttila E, Paajanen H, Turula A (2004) Extending a multimedia medical record to a regional service including experiences with electronic referral and discharge letters. In: Proceedings of 4th international conference on successes and failures in telehealth, Brisbane, Journal of Telemedicine and Telecare, (Suppliment) p 23–24

18. Reponen J, Niinimäki J, Kumpulainen T, Ilkko E, Karttunen A, Jartti P (2005) Mobile teleradiology with smartphone terminals as a part of a multimedia electronic patient record. In: Lemke HU, Inamura K, Doi K, Vannier MW, Farman AG (eds) Proceedings of CARS 2005. Elsevier, Berlin, pp 916–921

19. Reponen J, Winblad I, Hamalainen P, Kangas M (2006) Status of digital radiology image archiving and transfer in Finnish hospital districts. In: Doupi P, Winblad I, Reponen J (eds) Proceeding of the 6th Nordic conference on eHealth & telemedicine, NCeHT2006, 31 August–1 September 2006, TUCS Publications, Finlandia Hall, Helsinki, Finland. pp 49–50
20. Tervonen O (2007) Kuinka vaikuttaa radiologian toimintaan (How to influence radiological services). In: Proceedings of the 12th Finnish national conference on telemedicine and eHealth, 26–27 April 2007, TUCS Publications Kuopio, Finland
21. Wootton R, Harno K, Reponen J (2003) Organizational aspects of e-referrals. J Telemed Telecare, WSOY Publisher, 9(Suppl 2):S76–S79

Wireless Teleradiology and Security

Ayis T. Pyrros and Vahid Yaghmai

Abstract A basic overview of wireless networks and radiology applications of wireless teleradiology networks is given. Also, security of wireless teleradiology networks is scrutinized.

18.1
Introduction

Teleradiology offers clinicians and radiologists alike the ability to view diagnostic radiology images virtually anywhere, with almost any type of computer device [14]. This flexibility has prompted clinicians and radiologists alike to explore freedoms in viewing imaging remotely and locally, without the chains of restrictive computer wires. Where it was once necessary to have physical copies of radiographs, it is now possible to have the radiologist and clinician simultaneously view images great distances apart or in the hospital setting without even so much as a plug in sight [10]. Teleradiology has grown rapidly, with Larson et al. [8] finding that 75% of radiologists with multiple practices and 30% of solo radiologists started using teleradiology in 1999. The possibilities are exciting; however, many new complexities arise from the use of such technology [15]. This chapter will cover the basics of wireless teleradiology, including advantages and disadvantages of the technology compared with traditional methods of wired teleradiology.

18.2
Overview of Wireless Teleradiology

Wireless teleradiology is identical to teleradiology, with the obvious difference of using a radiofrequency wireless network for the digital communication of radiographic images. There are four major disadvantages with wireless technologies: reliability, cost, security, and speed. The obvious major advantage of such technology is the ability to view images virtually anywhere, from a patient's hospital room to the quagmire of the battlefield. In addition, in the last several years, the cost of wireless networks and their speed have become insignificant issues; in fact, many would argue that there is cost savings in deploying a wireless network, which does not require the expense of cabling [14].

18.3
Introduction to Wireless Networks

Modern technology is evolving with breakneck speed, and wireless networks are no exception. From a relative novelty 5 years ago, their presence is now ubiquitous. New deployments are increasing at a staggering rate, with almost all corporate laptop computers ready for shipping being wireless [16].

In the USA, the Health Insurance Portability and Accountability Act placed new standards on securing a patient's confidential medical information. This has brought the issue of information compliance to the forefront of the medical field, previously of major concern predominantly in the financial industry. Substantial penalties have been put in place to ensure compliance; the US Department of Health and Human Services has the authority to apply both civil and criminal penalties in the event of noncompliance [9].

The securing of wireless networks presents an additional challenge to the security of a network. Unlike wired networks, which are protected by physical contact to a wire or fiber-optic cable, wireless networks use radio waves. With standard antennas, these can transmit for several hundred meters, and, with modified antennas, distances as great as several kilometers have been recorded [6]. There is nothing to prevent anyone from eavesdropping on these signals, with nothing more than an appropriately equipped laptop. Not only can financial and other personal data be stolen, intruders can obtain protected patient information, thereby exposing the institution to legal liabilities. In addition to passively listening to network transmissions, criminals can, and do, use Wi-Fi to gain access to local or other networks via the Internet. When the investigating bodies trace the source of the illicit activity, the compromised wireless network is identified as the cause, despite the innocence of the actual network owner. Furthermore, leveraging security weaknesses in computer server operating systems, the unauthorized party may have the opportunity to willfully modify the data within, or prevent the function of, any information systems it is able to compromise. The potential for abuse is extensive and cannot be overemphasized.

18.4
Wireless Ethernet Standards

The seeds of wireless Ethernet were planted in 1985 when the Federal Communications Commission (FCC) made several bands of wireless spectrum available for unlicensed use [1]. Further changes to the FCC rules were made in 1989, enabling the future of Wi-Fi [1]. These frequencies at 900 MHz, 2.4 GHz, and 5.8 GHz were referred to as the "garbage bands" [1]. These frequencies were already in use, by devices like microwave ovens. Vendors in the late 1980s began to develop their own proprietary wireless technologies when they took interest into developing a standard wireless network protocol.

In 1988, the Institute of Electrical and Electronics Engineers (IEEE) founded a committee called 802.11 [1]. By September 1999, two standards had been ratified: 802.11b (operating at 2.4 GHz) and 802.11a (operating at 5.8 GHz) [1]. Soon after the 802.11 standard had been developed, the Wi-Fi Alliance trade group, based in Austin, Texas, USA, was created, which owns the trademark to Wi-Fi. The Wi-Fi Alliance is now responsible for the development of wireless standards. Early equipment suffered from issues of incompatibility, which were eventually resolved with testing. Today, the Wi-Fi logo ensures that the device being purchased will function on a wireless network.

Wireless networking products took hold with home consumers because of the popularity of effortlessly sharing an Internet connection without the hassle of cables. Over the next several years, wireless networking technology began to find its place in the corporate environment.

An 802.11b network transmits at 2.4 GHz and sends data at speeds up to 11 Mbps using direct sequence spread spectrum modulation. However, the 2.4 GHz spectrum is crowded with signals from other devices, such as cordless phones and microwave ovens, and other networks such as Bluetooth™. Bluetooth™ is a short-range network designed to quickly connect electronic devices such as cellular or mobile phones, headsets, cameras, and printers.

An 802.11a radio transmits at 5.8 GHz and sends data at speeds up to 54 Mbps, using orthogonal frequency division multiplexing (OFDM). Although the 5 GHz spectrum is less crowded than the 2.4 GHz spectrum, its signals have a higher absorption rate, resulting in signal loss through walls and objects. More recently, 802.11 g was released, which operates in the 2.4 GHz spectrum using OFDM, achieving theoretical speeds up to 54 Mbps [4].

When wireless Ethernet was developed, little emphasis was given to security. The first priority was interoperability between various hardware vendors. The first security standard, known as wired equivalent privacy (WEP), was developed in late 1997 [6]. Many vendors did not implement WEP initially [17]. By 2001, it was well documented that WEP itself was insecure [6]. A replacement encryption standard, Wi-Fi protected access (WPA), did not become available until late 2002 [17]. Ultimately, it was not until September 2003 that WPA security became a requirement for Wi-Fi certification [17].

18.5
Mobile Network Standards

Similar to Wi-Fi, most mobile devices offer the ability to transmit images through standard mobile networks. In the USA, several technologies, each of which is proprietary to the operator, exist, such as code division multiple access (CDMA) and GSM. The worldwide standard is GSM. There is an obvious cost of using such networks, but they can provide access even in some of the most remote areas. However, they typically offer data transmission speeds that are significantly slower than those of Wi-Fi. Furthermore, although such networks are encrypted, multiple studies have demonstrated them to be insecure and vulnerable.

18.6
Importance of Wireless Teleradiology

There are obvious conveniences associated with wireless technologies in everyday life; but can they be applied to radiology? Kim et al. [7] demonstrated that the mobility and portability from the use of a personal digital assistant (PDA) in the emergency setting were helpful without requiring the consultant to be in a fixed location. They also found that using a CBMA 1×-Evolution Data-Only network (cellular network) was adequate for rapid transmission of images.

Beyond the use of rapid interpretation, Yaghmai et al. [20] found that cellular networks were helpful in distributing teaching file cases to education radiology residents on away rotations. The time from receipt of an e-mail to the viewing of the images was less than 20 s for all cases. The images were all of diagnostic image quality. These examples show that in a world of instant access, wireless devices are a near necessity to keep pace.

18.7
Applications of Wireless Teleradiology

Since the ratification and widespread development of the 802.11 standard, Wi-Fi networks have progressively become cheaper and faster. There are unlimited numbers of applications for wireless technologies and teleradiology. In this section, we will attempt to discuss a select few case examples.

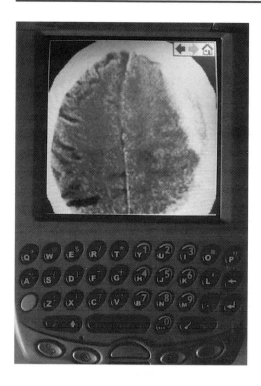

Fig. 18.1. A subdural hematoma with midline shift on a wireless personal digital assistant. (Used with permission from Vahid Yaghmai)

One of the simplest methods by which wireless teleradiology may be implemented is using a PDA and a built-in digital camera (Fig. 18.1). PDAs have evolved from a relative novelty to full-fledged computing workhorses in less than 20 years [5]. Today's PDA is closer to an ultraportable laptop than a simple personal information manager, with the ability to handle multimedia and access gigabytes of data [5]. Additionally, it offers portability in a form factor that easily fits into a pocket or laboratory coat [5].

Today's built-in camera phones have standard resolutions of about two megapixels, which is more than adequate for the capture and transmission of a single image. The image can be acquired from a light box or even a standard picture archiving and communication system monitor with the appropriate lighting conditions [21]. The image can then be sent using standard simple mail transport protocol, which is typically included on most PDA devices as an e-mail client. The images are typically compressed in a lossy image format such as Joint Photographic Experts Group (JPEG) format and encoded for transmission through e-mail. The limiting factors of acquiring the image through a digital camera are a less than perfect capture of the image and the relatively time consuming process of taking pictures for each image one wishes to transmit. In addition, this method is insecure, and identifying patient information should not be included on the image.

Reponen et al. [11] demonstrated that PDAs equipped with GSM wireless network capability can be useful in transmitting images of small examinations to allow for prompt diagnosis. The study focused on sending computed tomography examination images to a neuroradiologist. There was a significant delay of approximately 21 min in sending the entire examination images, with transmission of a single image requiring 1.5 min.

Additional work done by Yaghmai et al. [19] found that PDAs are an effective way to transmit 256×256 pixel resolution images through a PDA using CDMA wireless network. These images were sent through standard e-mail clients, using a standard commercially available Treo-270 communicator PDA (palmOne, Milpitas, CA, USA). Since the time of these studies, PDAs have continued to advance with faster processors and wireless network connections, increased storage capabilities, and improved screen resolutions. The recently released Apple iPhone (Caperunico, CA, USA) has an impressive screen resolution of 480×320 pixels with Wi-Fi capability. In addition, almost all PDAs now offer the ability to connect to standard Wi-Fi networks, in addition to standard cellular networks. These portable devices will only continue to improve.

In using a PDA, both Yaghmai et al. and Reponen et al. discussed the limitations of viewing a large number of images over the relatively slow speeds of a GSM and CDMA phone network. The relatively small screen size and slow speed of a PDA add additional limitations in viewing the images from large complex radiological studies. Interestingly, recent research demonstrates that compressing thin-section images using JPEG 2000 noticeably increases the noise of the image [18]. In fact, a lower compression for thin-section abdominal computed tomography images or alternatively thicker sections may be needed [18].

In addition to using standard CDMA and Wi-Fi, other wireless technologies such as Bluetooth⁻ may be employed for the transmission of images over a short distance [7]. This provides the added convenience of wireless communication over a short distance that could be used in a hospital inpatient setting. Kim et al. [7] advocated that such a system allows for "synchronized radiological image sharing."

18.8
Wireless Security Overview

Wireless security generally has three goals: (1) to restrict wireless access to authorized users, (2) to restrict which devices are allowed access to the host network, and (3) to encrypt wireless data transmission to prevent eavesdropping, modification, or insertion of data with respect to the wireless data stream. Server and client security (including personal computers, PCs; laptops; PDAs; etc.) is a separate, but equally important, security objective.

The difficulty with security, in general, is that it is a moving target. What is considered "very secure" today will be considered "extremely insecure" within a finite amount of time. Security "best practices" are ever changing; it is critical to keep up with evolving threats. Exploits of breaking computer security are disseminated online very quickly. As a general caveat, no network is 100% secure, and it is necessary to include the costs of regular updates in any network or wireless budgets.

"Best practices" are methods and procedures generally accepted by the leaders in their field as the best techniques to accomplish a particular goal. The technology field's use of the term "best practices" is analogous to the medical term "evidence-based medicine."

18.9
Hacking the Network

Besides compromised encryption, wireless networks are susceptible to other forms of attack. A denial of service attack bombards a wireless access point with useless information packets that can overwhelm a wireless network, rendering it useless. Man in the middle, or TCP hijacking, is another well-documented attack in which a wireless transmission can be intercepted between the access point and the client (laptops, PDAs, and workstations) [3]. Malicious association involves the creation of a new access point and deceiving clients' computers to associate with it, in order to break into the client computer. In fact, a user may accidentally join the incorrect network, transmitting potentially sensitive data to the wrong location [13].

WEP was the first widely used wireless encryption standard deployed. The standard has since been compromised and is now considered insecure. The primary weakness with WEP is that it is based on a single shared static key, used for both decryption and encryption (a symmetric key) (Fig. 18.2). WEP today is deployed with 64- and 128-bit keys, the 128-bit key offering more security with an increased number of key combinations. All clients and devices use the same key in order to communicate with the access point (Fig. 18.3). Once a key is compromised, the attacker can decrypt and read all wireless network traffic until the symmetric key is changed for all communicating parties. Unfortunately, within the WEP standard there is no automated mechanism to enforce length of key life and change keys.

Numerous decryption attacks against WEP have been developed to take advantage of its weak encryption algorithm. These decryption attacks have been automated and simplified by software packages that are freely available on the Internet. A typical attack records wireless Ethernet traffic to and from the access point, analyzes the information, and determines a key.

A decryption attack using a popular software package called Aircrack needs approximately 24 h to break a 128-bit WEP key and requires only five million to

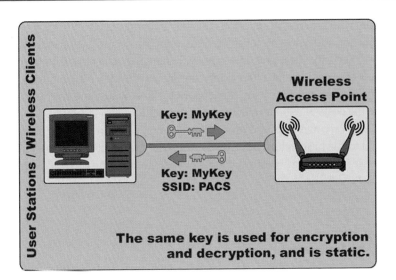

Fig. 18.2. The weakness of wired equivalent privacy (WEP), which uses a static (nonchanging) encryption key. WEP is unsafe and should not be used to transmit confidential patient information

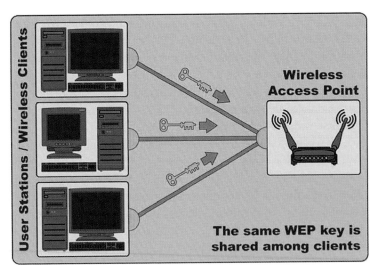

Fig. 18.3. An additional weakness of WEP encryption is the same key (or password) is shared by multiple computers. Therefore, if security is compromised on a single computer, it is compromised for all computers on the wireless network

ten million encrypted packets to be gathered. Once enough information packets have been gathered, Aircrack can guess the encryption password in under 1 s [2]. Walker's [22] paper "Unsafe at any key length" says it all in the title. Papers from the University of California at Berkley and the University of Maryland also showed the weaknesses of WEP. Unfortunately, older wireless routers and wireless cards only offer WEP as an encryption protocol. The best solution is to upgrade the hardware. Other attacks use a combination of dictionary methods, mathematics, and known encryption weaknesses. It may be wise to consider dynamically generated passwords for sensitive data, in addition to nonpassword methods of authentication such as biometrics.

Lightweight extensible authentication protocol (LEAP) is Cisco Systems's (Cisco Systems, San Jose, CA, USA) proprietary implementation of extensible authentication protocol (EAP), and it requires all Cisco hardware including wireless Ethernet adapters and access points. LEAP provides dynamically changing keys during sessions. It was one of the first more popular alternatives to WEP. It is commonly used in hospital networks today. However, LEAP has vulnerabilities in the way passwords are handled (passing them as unencrypted text) and has been shown to be susceptible to dictionary attacks. Password-based authentication algorithms are vulnerable to dictionary attacks. During such an attack, an intruder tries to guess a user's password in order to gain network access by using every single word from a dictionary of common passwords or potential combinations of passwords. It takes advantage of the fact that passwords most often comprise common words, names, or in many instances common words or names with a minor modification such as a subsequent number (such as Paul72). Again, longer passwords with a variety of characters (such as g7u18sccP) offer the greatest protection against dictionary attacks.

Protected extensible authentication protocol (PEAP) was based on an Internet draft written by Cisco Systems, Microsoft (Redmond, WA, USA) and RSA Security (, Bedford, MA, USA). It provides enhanced security by employing key encryption management; this requires the additional hardware and software of an authentication server. An authentication server is a dedicated server responsible for the management and security of user keys. PEAP encrypts all client and authentication server communications, unlike LEAP. Unfortunately, this standard has also been compromised and is insecure.

18.10
Securing the Network

A typical computer network is composed of clients (laptops, PDAs, and workstations) and servers, with hubs and routers acting as communication nexus points. Wireless access points typically come as a combined switched hub (allowing 10 and 100 Mbit wired Ethernet speeds) and a router. The anatomy of a wireless network requires that any point of access to the network be secure. Devices may include file servers, PDAs, laptops, or workstations that have a wireless Internet interface and connect to a wireless network. An insecure or compromised wireless station can become a launch pad to breach the entire network. For instance, a laptop that is infected with spyware or keylogging software can monitor and transmit user activity. This software is oftentimes installed without the user's knowledge. This software may also send secure passwords and information that can allow easy access to a network or server. Therefore, clients must be well secured (current patches, firewall, antivirus, antispyware, and tough-to break passwords); however, discussion of this is beyond the scope of this paper. Please see http://www.nsa.gov/snac for current security configuration guidelines.

18.11
Secure the Access Point

The security of a wireless network must first begin with the wireless access point. Despite the wide number of different wireless routers available, their setup and configuration methods are remarkably similar. Most routers offer an easy-access Web-based configuration utility, usually accessed through a Web browser with a default IP address. In addition, each router is shipped with a default password for the configuration utility of the access point. With little effort, an intruder can gain access to the router by using known default access methods. Once access has been gained, the intruder may choose to modify security settings, disable access for others, and attempt to access other networks. It is therefore critical to (1) change the default password using a large combination of letters and numbers that is not easily guessable and (2) restrict administrative access to the wireless router through hard-wired Ethernet locations.

18.12
Service Set Identifier

As a part of the 802.11 standard, every wireless access point has the ability to broadcast its name, or service set identifier (SSID), which allows users the ability to easily locate a wireless access point. Generally, most wireless access points have the SSID broadcast enabled as a factory default. Generic titles such as wireless, linksys, and dlink are often seen. Even worse, some companies broadcast attractive names, such as finance-dept, as their SSID name. Although it does not restrict access, disabling SSID broadcasts can decrease the visibility of your wireless network to unwanted users.

18.13
Media Access Control Lists

Media access control (MAC) lists are another way to restrict wireless network access. A MAC address is a 48-bit number that is uniquely assigned to every network interface card by the manufacturer. The network administrator configures a list of authorized MAC addresses in each access point, or on the access server, thereby restricting access to the network to those specific MAC addresses (Fig. 18.4). However, unwanted users (hackers) may manually reconfigure their MAC address, thereby circumventing the table. Additionally, a MAC address is easily obtained by wireless eavesdropping. In any case, use of the MAC table is a further obstacle to unauthorized access.

18.14
Encryption

As previously discussed, WEP is not a secure standard and its use is not recommended. WPA was ratified in June 2003, and it is backward compatible with WEP, although this is self-defeating. WEP should be turned completely off. WPA provides relativity higher security than previous standards and is based on 802.1X EAP for authentication. WPA offers the option of both an

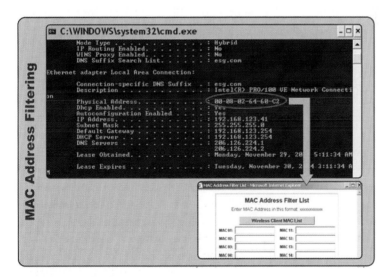

Fig. 18.4. A simple method to secure any network is to use media access control (*MAC*) addresses, which serve as unique identifiers of network interface cards. Unfortunately, it is relatively easy to change and duplicate MAC addresses

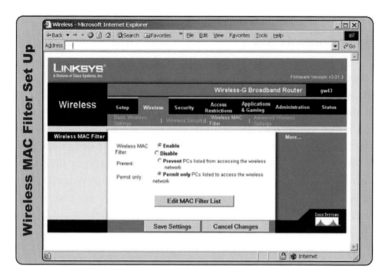

Wireless MAC Filter Set Up

Fig. 18.5. Newer wireless routers provide advanced encryption methods such as advanced encryption standard and Wi-Fi protected access

authentication server model (enterprise mode) and a personal mode that does not require an additional authentication. Limitations of WPA include slower performance, in general, and a more complex setup. Some of its implementations also have vulnerabilities.

WPA2 is the most recently ratified standard. Based on the final IEEE 802.11i amendment to the 802.11 standard, it supports better key security with advanced encryption standard (Fig. 18.5). It is also compliant with the US government security standard FIPS140-2. New hardware compatible with WPA2 is just now being introduced onto the market. In order for new products to be certified as Wi-Fi, they must be WPA2-compliant.

WPA encryption with very long and complex passwords is probably the best Wi-Fi security one can install today. One should be prepared, however, to convert to WPA2 as equipment becomes available.

18.15
Layered Security

A multilayered approach greatly reduces the risk of a compromised network. Virtual private network (VPN) gateways between the wireless local-area network (WLAN) and the wired network offer further security. Unauthorized and legitimate users could attach to the WLAN alike, but only authenticated users would be able to pass traffic through the gateway via the VPN. In addition, encrypted tunnels such as Secure Sockets Layer and IP security (IPSec) use far stronger encryption than WEP and are difficult to break in most circumstances [12].

The first step in layering security is to isolate the Wi-Fi connection to a dedicated network segment. Then, one would use a VPN gateway to connect the Wi-Fi network and the corporate network. This is considered a "best practice" for good wireless security. Even in the event that the Wi-Fi network is compromised, damages are limited. The intruder would have to expend further resources to compromise the VPN gateway, or compromise the wireless network PCs/PDAs, in order to access the internal network or other data.

18.16
Other Measures

It is sensible for additional layers of network security to be implemented wherever practical. Additional measures to provide network security include disabling wireless access during nonbusiness hours and implementing secure server rooms (which physically protects hardware from tampering). Wireless networks need to be monitored constantly for evidence of tampering or intrusion. Software companies offer passive monitoring systems that help detect attackers. Regular information technology audits, performed by a third party, should be considered a standard part of any company's management procedures. Intrusion detection systems can monitor systems for any breach and sound an alarm should one occur.

In summary, a strong, multilayered approach is the most effective means we have today to mitigate the risk posed by a wireless network. This approach includes the application of "best practices," audits, and regular updates throughout all levels of the information systems involved.

Wireless encryption standards will continue to evolve; therefore, it is imperative to include realistic hardware upgrade and maintenance costs in all information technology budgets.

WiMAX technology (IEEE standard 802.16) will provide long-distance wireless connectivity. This will enable wireless deployments on city-wide scales, without use of phone lines, lasers, or other expensive interconnections.

18.17
Conclusions

In turn, wireless access to teleradiology systems will be seamless. Availability of a remote physician consultant should improve patient care by rapid access to distant subspecialists. Although, wireless teleradiology is in its infancy and its security is a prime concern when transmitting patient data, the present technology offers significant possibilities for improved patient care.

Summary

Important points discussed in the chapter are summarized as follows:

- Basic overview of wireless networks
- Radiology applications of wireless teleradiology networks
- Security of wireless teleradiology networks

References

1. Anonymous (2004) A brief history of Wi-Fi. Economist, p 8
2. www.aircrack-ng.org. Last Accessed 29 April 2008
3. Definition of man-in-the-middle (2002). www.bsacybersafety.com. Last Accessed 29 April 2008
4. Ferrante FE (2006) Maintaining security and privacy of patient information. Conf Proc IEEE Eng Med Biol Soc 1:4690
5. Flanders AE, Wiggins RH III, Gozum ME (2003) Handheld computers in radiology. Radiographics 23(4):1035–1047
6. Gast M (2002) Wireless LAN security: a short history. Wirelss Devcenter. www.oreillynet.com/pub/a/wireless/2002/04/19/security.html. Last Accessed 29 April 2008
7. Kim DK, Yoo SK, Park JJ, Kim SH (2007) PDA-phone-based instant transmission of radiological images over a CDMA network by combining the PACS screen with a Bluetooth-interfaced local wireless link. J Digit Imaging 20(2):131–139
8. Larson DB CY, Forman HP, Sunshine JH (2005) A comprehensive portrait of teleradiology in radiology practices: results from the American College of Radiology's 1999 survey. AJR Am J Roentgenol 185:24–25
9. Office for Civil Rights (2005) Privacy of health records
10. Puech PA, Boussel L, Belfkih S, Lemaitre L, Douek P, Beuscart R (2007) DicomWorks: software for reviewing DICOM studies and promoting low-cost teleradiology. J Digit Imaging 20(2):122–130
11. Reponen J, Ilkko E, Jyrkinen L et al (2000) Initial experience with a wireless personal digital assistant as a teleradiology terminal for reporting emergency computerized tomography scans. J Telemed Telecare 6(1):45–49
12. (2000) Step-by-step guide to Internet protocol security (IPSec) Microsoft Technet. http://technet.microsoft.com/en-us/library/bb742429.aspx. Last Accessed 29 April 2008
13. Risks dig 23(16) (1988) The Risks Digest http://catless.ncl.ac.uk/Risks/7.23.html. Last Accessed 29 April 2008
14. Thrall JH (2007) Teleradiology. Part I. History and clinical applications. Radiology 243(3):613–617
15. Thrall JH (2007) Teleradiology. Part II. Limitations, risks, and opportunities. Radiology 244(2):325–328

16. (2003) 95 Percent of notebooks to have wireless capabilities by 2005. Wireless Advis March 2003 www.qualcomm.com/enterprise/pdf/Embedded_CDMANotebook.pdf. Last Accessed 29 April 2008

17. (2003) Wireless LAN time line. PC Mag. www.pcmag.com/article2/0,1759,1276145,00. asp. Last Accessed 29 April 2008

18. Woo HS, Kim KJ, Kim TJ et al (2007) JPEG 2000 compression of abdominal CT: difference in tolerance between thin- and thick-section images. AJR Am J Roentgenol 189(3):535–541

19. Yaghmai V, Salehi SA, Kuppuswami S, Berlin JW (2004) Rapid wireless transmission of head CT images to a personal digital assistant for remote consultation. Acad Radiol 11(11):1291–1293

20. Yaghmai VKR, Pyrros A, Rohany M, Casalino D (2005) Feasibility of using a wireless PDA to distribute teaching files to radiology residents in a large teaching institution with several teaching sites. RSNA, Chicago

21. Yamada M, Watarai H, Andou T, Sakai N (2003) Emergency image transfer system through a mobile telephone in Japan: technical note. Neurosurgery 52(4):986–988; discussion 988–990

22. Walker JR (2000) Unsafe at any key size; an analysis of the WEP encapsulation. IEEE P802.11 wireless LANs 2000; IEEE 802.11-00/362.

19

High-Volume Teleradiology Service: Focus on Radiologist and Patient Satisfaction

Elizabeth A. Krupinski

Abstract Increased display luminance, use of a P45 (rather than a P104) phosphor in the cathode ray tube monitor faceplate, and a perceptually linearized display lead to better diagnostic accuracy and more efficient visual search. For radiology as well as teleradiology, the viewing workstation is crucial. Spending long hours viewing very large data sets on computer screens may result in visual fatigue or computer vision syndrome among radiologists, leading to dissatisfaction among them. Teleradiology, telepathology, and teleoncology together can be used to reduce the waiting times for breast cancer patients to receive definitive care and increase significant patient satisfaction and general peace of mind.

19.1
Introduction

Teleradiology is probably the oldest and most successful telemedicine application being practiced today. In large part, this is due to the inherently digital nature of the images used (or ease with which film images can be converted to a digital format), the widespread implementation of picture archiving and communications systems, and the fact that the radiologists did not have to alter significantly their diagnostic task or interpretation procedure. With both hard-copy and soft-copy formats, the radiologist views an image and renders a diagnostic decision. In most clinical situations, this takes place off-line (i.e., the patient does not have direct contact with the radiologist and the image is generally interpreted after the patient leaves), and with teleradiology the same is true. This chapter will cover the following points, using the teleradiology program at the University of Arizona as an example program:

- Factors that contribute to dissatisfaction of the radiologists
- Factors that contribute to improved image quality
- The relation between soft-copy viewing of images and radiologist fatigue
- A unique telemammography program

The Arizona Telemedicine Program (ATP) was created in 1996 by the Arizona State Legislature as a multidisciplinary, university-based program to provide telemedicine services, distance learning, informatics training, and telemedicine technology assessment throughout the state of Arizona. The Legislature mandated that the program provide telemedicine services to a broad range of health-care service users, including geographically isolated communities, Indian tribes, and the Department of Corrections. Following an initial implementation in 1997 with eight pilot sites, the ATP now operates a broadband telecommunications network that links over 150 not-for-profit and profit health-care organizations, functioning as a "virtual corporation." The core mission of the ATP is to provide access to specialty health-care services for medically underserved communities in the rural areas of the state.

Our teleradiology network (managed by the ATP) uses a scalable T-1/asynchronous transfer mode broadband telecommunication system, which connects over 150 sites around the state of Arizona [16]. The network is used for a variety of telemedicine-related activities, including clinical, educational, and administrative. Teleradiology represents the most common use of the network, with over 100,000 cases transmitted per year in recent years. The teleradiology program began in 1996 and, as Fig. 19.1 shows, has grown considerably since then. The Department of Radiology at the University of Arizona currently provides interpretation services to 33 sites around the state in both rural and urban areas. We cover most modalities including computed radiography, digital radiography, computed tomography, ultrasound, magnetic resonance imaging, fluoroscopy, mammography, nuclear medicine (single proton emission computed tomography and positron emission tomography), and angiography (Fig. 19.2). Echocardiography interpretation services are also provided through the Department of Cardiology for both adult and pediatric patients using real-time echocardiography techniques.

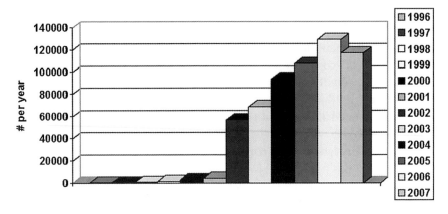

Fig. 19.1. Number of teleradiology cases interpreted each year since the program began in 1996. Note that 2007 only includes cases through August 2007

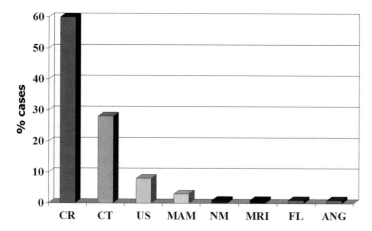

Fig. 19.2. Percentage of cases interpreted in each modality since the teleradiology program began in 1996. *CR* computed radiography, *CT* computed tomography, *US* ultrasound, *MAM* mammography, *NM* nuclear medicine, *MRI* magnetic resonance imaging, *FL* fluoroscopy, *ANG* angiography

19.1.1
Factors that contribute to dissatisfaction of the radiologists

When the program first began in 1996, we asked our radiologists about the program as a measure of quality control and satisfaction [10]. Many of the questions dealt with how many teleradiology cases they had read and what types, but we also asked them about image quality. At that time (1998), 63% of the radiologists reported that the images had excellent or very good quality and 90% rated the user-friendliness of the workstation as excellent or good. That question was followed by asking if they felt their diagnostic confidence was the same as, better than, or worse than with traditional film reading. Forty-two percent said that their confidence was the same and 68% percent said it was lower. When asked what factors reduced their confidence in their diagnostic decisions, 71% said it was because of poor image quality—specifically digitized images that they could not window/level very well. Not having a clinical history was the second most common reason (14.5% of respondents), followed by not having enough images (especially priors) as reported by 14.5% of the respondents. Because of this study we changed our policy regarding the types of images we would accept for teleradiology. If a site wanted to send plain film images (chest, abdomen, and bone for the most part), it would have to invest in a computed radiography system so that images could be acquired digitally and sent in that digital format. Although it was a financial investment, all sites connected to the network for teleradiology services now use digital acquisition systems. The radiologists have expressed little to no concern with image quality since then.

19.1.2
Factors that contribute to improved image quality

Another aspect of image quality that is absolutely crucial to accurate interpretation and user satisfaction is the display. We have carried out a number of studies to characterize digital displays and optimize their display properties. Early efforts focused on comparing film with soft-copy displays, with emphasis on measuring diagnostic accuracy and visual search behaviors as measured using eye-position recording techniques [4, 7, 8, 15]. Once soft-copy viewing was established as being comparable to hard-copy viewing, we began examining various physical properties of monitors to determine whether they influence diagnostic accuracy and visual search efficiency. We started with cathode ray tube (CRT) displays and then moved to liquid crystal displays. We found that increased display luminance [11], use of a P45 (rather than a P104) phosphor in the CRT monitor faceplate [6, 13], and a perceptually linearized (i.e., with the digital imaging and communications in medicine standard rather than a non-perceptually linearized) display [5] lead to better diagnostic accuracy and more efficient visual search. Efficient visual search is characterized by shorter times to first fixate a lesion in the image with foveal vision early in the search, shorter overall dwell times on lesions (with better detection), and shorter total viewing times. We have also looked at the effectiveness and use of image processing [9, 12] and the role reader experience plays in the interpretation of medical images [2, 8, 15]. In terms of image processing, it seems that different radiologists prefer different processing tools. For example, some radiologists will use the edge-enhancement feature on all images before they even begin their search for lesions. Others will use little to no processing at all. The use of zoom and pan is just as idiosyncratic.

More recently, we have started to investigate the use of color monitors in teleradiology. A number of radiologists prefer to work at home now that high-speed secure connections to personal residences are relatively inexpensive. Although the telecommunications side of teleradiology has become quite affordable, the cost of high-performance monochrome displays that are generally used in the clinic has not decreased significantly. Teleradiologists would prefer to use color monitors that can be purchased off the shelf at a more reasonable cost. Therefore, we evaluated the clinical utility for teleradiology of a high-performance (3 megapixel) color display compared with that of two monochrome displays—one of comparable luminance (250 cd/m^2) and one of higher luminance (450 cd/m^2) [14]. Six radiologists viewed 50 chest images, half with nodules and half without, on each display. We recorded their eye position on a subset of the images to study visual search efficiency (Fig. 19.3).

We found no statistically significant difference in diagnostic performance as a function of monitor ($F = 1.176$, $p = 0.3127$), although the higher-luminance

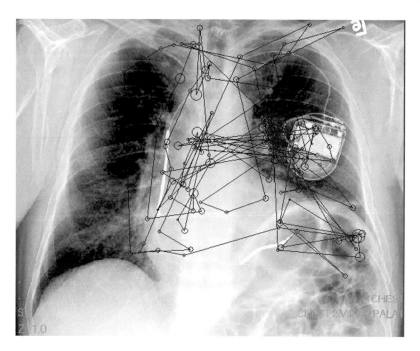

Fig. 19.3. Typical eye-position pattern of a radiologist searching a chest image for pulmonary nodules. Each *circle* represents a fixation or location where the high-resolution foveal part of the eye lands. The size of the circle indicates the dwell time, with larger circles representing longer dwell. The lines indicate the order in which the fixations were generated

monochrome display was slightly better. For total viewing time, there were no statistically significant differences between the monitors ($F = 1.478$, $p = 0.2298$). The dwell times associated with true- and false-positive decisions were shortest for the high-luminance monochrome display and longest for the low-luminance color display. Dwells for the false-negative decisions were longest for the high-luminance monochrome display and shortest for the low-luminance color display. The true-negative dwells were not different. The study suggests that high-performance color displays can be used for teleradiologic interpretation of diagnostic images without negatively impacting diagnostic accuracy or visual search efficiency.

19.1.3
The relation between softcopy viewing of images and radiologist fatigue

For radiology in general, as well as for teleradiology, the viewing workstation is crucial [3]. The display, however, is not the only consideration. The input device, although generally a matter of personal preference, is important

Table 19.1. Subjective visual fatigue symptoms correlated with reading time and number of examinations radiologists read

Symptom	Reading time	Number of examinations
Blurry vision	$R = 0.34, p < 0.02$	$R = 0.42, p < 0.002$
Eyestrain	$R = 0.43, p < 0.002$	$R = 0.48, p < 0.001$
Focus problems	$R = 0.38, p < 0.005$	$R = 0.45, p < 0.001$
Headache	$R = 0.24, p = 0.09$	$R = 0.43, p < 0.002$

to consider when looking at the radiologist's satisfaction with the teleradiology reading environment. Keyboards, mice, and track balls are the common input devices, but foot pedals, joysticks, modified keyboard/mouse combinations, and even voice-controlled technologies should be considered for improved user comfort. The risk of carpal tunnel syndrome and other repetitive musculoskeletal injuries for radiologists is not insignificant, so radiologists should choose an input device that they are physically comfortable with.

One concern with digital displays in radiology and teleradiology that has not been considered very much is visual fatigue or computer vision syndrome. This may result from the long hours that radiologists spend viewing very large data sets every day on computer screens. This could, in turn, lead to dissatisfaction with reading conditions and possibly even general job dissatisfaction among radiologists. As a first step in finding out whether fatigue is an important problem in the radiology reading room, we created a short survey to evaluate fatigue of radiologists at different times during the day. The survey asked about symptoms of visual and postural fatigue, the types and number of cases they had been interpreting, and total reading time that day. We gave the survey to radiologists and residents in the morning and afternoon over a number of days. Table 19.1 shows correlations between the number of cases, reading time, and reported symptoms of fatigue.

We saw a significant positive correlation between the time reading cases and the severity of the visual fatigue symptoms. There was a trend toward higher fatigue when radiologists view both film and digitally displayed images on the same day. Film-only reading gave the lowest fatigue ratings, followed by digital-only reading. Clearly, radiologists are becoming fatigued as they view more and more images on digital displays, and the only way to view teleradiology cases is using soft-copy presentation.

19.1.4
A unique telemammography program

As noted above, telemammography accounts for about 3% of the total teleradiology volume in our program. The majority of these cases come from sites around the state with large Native American populations, including a number of Indian Health Service hospitals and clinics. Breast cancer is the most common cancer in women in the USA and around the world. In the USA, it is the second leading cause of cancer deaths in women [17]. Breast cancer is typically detected during screening using mammography and clinical breast examinations, and it is estimated that over 48 million mammograms are performed every year in the USA and the number is increasing. If something is detected on mammography and not resolvable by a diagnostic workup using magnified mammography views, spot imaging, ultrasound, or less frequently magnetic resonance imaging, a biopsy is performed. Fewer than one million (2–5%) women require a subsequent biopsy [18], and luckily the majority of biopsies (65–80%) result in benign diagnoses. However, malignancy is found in one in ten women who undergo breast biopsy [1]. In rural, medically underserved areas, mammography rates are generally lower for a variety of reasons, including lack of dedicated screening facilities and/or personnel, poor compliance, and large distances between patients and clinics (making it difficult to return for follow-up care). Telemammography has been found to alleviate significantly this problem in many rural areas, including those in Arizona.

We are starting to introduce a new program with telemammography at its core to further improve breast care for women. If breast cancer is detected, the process, from mammography to clinical consultation with the oncologist, usually takes about 28 days before treatment begins. If an abnormality is found, a diagnostic biopsy is performed at the mammography center or by a surgeon. The biopsied tissue is processed and then read by a pathologist, who generates a report and sends it back to the surgeon. A malignant diagnosis results in the patient scheduling a meeting with the medical oncologist for consultation and a treatment plan. This takes even longer for women in rural areas because they typically need to travel to an urban hospital for many of these procedures. Whether urban or rural, the long wait time between initial diagnosis, pathology results, and possibly oncology consultation can be extremely stressful for the patient. Teleradiology, telepathology, and teleoncology are ways that we are using to reduce the waiting times for a woman with breast cancer to receive definitive care.

On the telemammography side of the process, we have established contracts with the rural sites that specify a turnaround time (from receipt to generation and transmission of a report back to the site) of no more than 30 min for diagnostic cases and no more than 45 min for screening cases. We found over 90%

compliance with the turnaround times required in the service contracts at all sites. Discrepancies occurred mostly owing to transmission difficulties, not prolonged times once the images arrived at the interpretation workstation.

To incorporate the telepathology and teleoncology portions into the process, we have initiated ultrarapid breast clinics. The first study we did before setting up the process was to survey patients at the university breast clinic to determine if and how much women would be willing to pay for faster pathology results if they needed a biopsy. The willingness to pay for pathology services study had 312 responses. If diagnosed with cancer, 92% of the respondents in this study reported that they would seek a second expert opinion. The data were unevenly distributed ($\chi^2 = 51.14$, df $= 4$, $p < 0.001$), with 33% of the participants reporting a willingness to travel over 50 miles and 47% willing to travel between 11 and 50 miles. When asked if they would pay a copayment for a second opinion if their insurance covered the benefit, 97% of those surveyed responded affirmatively. Thirty-five percent of respondents reported that they would pay more than $50 for such a service. The distribution of values suggested that significantly more of the individuals surveyed would be willing to pay $25 or more than those willing to pay less than $25 ($\chi^2 = 139.52$, df $= 5$, $p < 0.0001$).

In another experiment, we studied whether digital scanning of pathology specimen slides to ensure that rapid processing and transmission for interpretation could be accomplished. For this we used the DMetrix virtual slide processor that samples images at 0.47 $\propto$m/pixel to scan a series of breast specimen images for interpretation on a computer display monitor and compared the interpretations with those made with the original slide images. Diagnostic accuracy and reading times were recorded. The study showed that diagnostic performance with the digital slides viewed on a computer display is equivalent to that resulting from viewing traditional slides ($\kappa > 0.90$ for all readers). The viewing times were significantly longer, although these are likely to decrease as better user interfaces are developed.

The final pilot study evaluated the teleoncology component. Patients needing a core biopsy were approached for participation. We followed the biopsy process. The tissue was processed by a vacuum histoprocess and ultrarapid fixation system, was converted to a digital image by the DMetrix scanner, and was then sent via the telemedicine network to be read via telepathology. The patient then went to the telemedicine suite to receive the results. The teleoncologist presented all results and all questions were answered. The time course of the entire process was recorded. The elapsed-time (from mammogram to definitive oncology care) data were analyzed comparing the control (patients receiving traditional care) and pilot groups (ultrarapid) using the nonparametric Mann–Whitney U test. Although the results did not reach statistical significance because of the very small sample size ($Z = -1.804$, $p = 0.0713$), there was a clear trend toward the pilot group having a shorter elapsed time to definitive oncology care. The median elapsed time for the pilot group was 2 months and for the control group was 2.5 months, with 3 months being the longest elapsed time for the pilot group and 5 months the longest for the control group.

On the basis of the results of these various pilot studies, we have started to offer these UltraClinics in hospitals in Tucson and are beginning to expand to rural areas as well. Early results suggest that the time saved via the telemammography, telepathology, and teleoncology procedures results in significant patient satisfaction and general peace of mind for those patients in whom normal results are found after an initial suspicious finding. Even for those patients for whom an abnormal finding is finally made, there is greater peace of mind owing to the rapid nature of the reporting process and the speed with which they are placed in contact with the oncologist who will be treating them. As a further step to helping these women in whom breast cancer is found, we are initiating telehelp groups. In many cases, women in rural areas have very few other women with breast cancer to whom they can turn for help, advice, and comfort. By connecting women in rural communities with each other via videoconferencing systems either in their homes or in local clinics, we hope to bridge these gaps in support.

In conclusion, we have been conducting teleradiology consultations for over 10 years in Arizona, within our Department of Radiology at the University of Arizona. Services, have expanded significantly over the years, and include a wide variety of modalities, including telemammography. Our radiologists are satisfied with the quality of the images received from the rural sites, and the rural sites are satisfied with the quality of reports they receive. Teleradiology has served as the foundation on which to build related services. Our telemammography program has expanded to include telepathology and teleoncology services to support the entire breast-care environment. As the ATP expands its network to more sites in the state of Arizona, our teleradiology services will continue to expand as well. Future telemedicine technologies, including remotely operated robotic systems, may even lead to the ability to do teleinterventional radiology, although these may be a few years in coming.

Summary

- Teleradiology is the oldest and most successful telemedicine application being practiced today.
- Increased display luminance, use of a P45 (rather than a P104) phosphor in the CRT monitor faceplate, and a perceptually linearized display lead to better diagnostic accuracy and more efficient visual search.
- For radiology as well as teleradiology, the viewing workstation is crucial. Spending long hours viewing very large data sets on computer screens may

result in visual fatigue or computer vision syndrome among radiologists, leading to dissatisfaction among them.

- Teleradiology, telepathology, and teleoncology together can be used to reduce the waiting times for breast cancer patients to receive definitive care and increase significant patient satisfaction and general peace of mind.

References

1. Imaginis—The Breast Health Resource (2005) Breast biopsy: indications and methods. http://imaginis.com/breasthealth/biopsy/#introduction. Accessed 26 Sep 2007
2. Krupinski EA (1996) Visual scanning patterns of radiologists searching mammograms. Acad Radiol 3:137–144
3. Krupinski EA, Kallergi M (2007) Choosing a radiology workstation: technical and clinical considerations. Radiology 242:671–682
4. Krupinski EA, Lund PJ (1997) Differences in time to interpretation for evaluation of bone radiographs with monitor and film viewing. Acad Radiol 4:177–182
5. Krupinski EA, Roehrig H (2000) The influence of a perceptually linearized display on observer performance and visual search. Acad Radiol 7:8–13
6. Krupinski EA, Roehrig H (2002) Pulmonary nodule detection and visual search: P45 and P104 monochrome versus color monitor displays. Acad Radiol 9:638–645
7. Krupinski EA, Maloney K, Bessen SC et al (1994) Receiver operating characteristic evaluation of computer display of adult portable chest radiographs. Invest Radiol 29:141–146
8. Krupinski EA, Weinstein RS, Rozek LS (1996) Experience-related differences in diagnosis from medical images displayed on monitors. Telemed J 2:101–108
9. Krupinski EA, Evanoff M, Ovitt T, Standen JR, Chu TX, Johnson J (1998) Influence of image processing on chest radiograph interpretation and decision changes. Acad Radiol 5:79–85
10. Krupinski EA, McNeill K, Ovitt TW, Alden S, Holcomb M (1999) Patterns of use and satisfaction with a university-based teleradiology system. J Digit Imaging 12:166–167
11. Krupinski E, Roehrig H, Furukawa T (1999) Influence of film and monitor display luminance on observer performance and visual search. Acad Radiol 6:411–418
12. Krupinski EA, Johnson JP, Roehrig H et al (2003) Using a human visual system model to optimize soft-copy mammography display: influence of MTF compensation. Acad Radiol 10:1030–1035
13. Krupinski EA, Johnson JP, Roehrig H, Lubin J (2003) Using a human visual system model to optimize soft-copy mammography display: influence of display phosphor. Acad Radiol 2003;10:161–166
14. Krupinski EA, Roehrig H, Fan J, Yoneda T (2007) High luminance monochrome vs low luminance monochrome and color softcopy displays: observer performance and visual search efficiency. Proc SPIE Med Imaging 6515:6515R-1
15. Lund PJ, Krupinski EA, Pereles S, Mockbee B (1997) Comparison of conventional and computed radiography: assessment of image quality and reader performance in skeletal extremity trauma. Acad Radiol 4:570–576
16. McNeill KM, Weinstein RS, Holcomb MJ (1998) Arizona Telemedicine Program: implementing a statewide care network. J Am Med Assoc 5:441–447
17. National Cancer Institute (2005) Breast cancer facts and figures. http://www.cancer.gov/cancertopics/types/breast. Accessed 26 Sep 2007
18. Susan G (2005) Komen Breast Cancer Foundation. About breast cancer: diagnosis and types of biopsies. http://www.komen.org/. Accessed 26 Sep 2007

20

Global Trade in Teleradiology: Economic and Legal Concerns

Thomas R. McLean and Patrick B. McLean

Abstract In the global market for teleradiology, a developing country has an absolute price advantage. However, opportunity costs and language skills will limit how much teleradiology a country can export. Better market regulation may be achieved by modification of the Internet's architecture or the commoditization of the market.

20.1
Introduction

Today, most teleradiology services are consumed in the country of their origin [31]. Yet, in the global market two separate models for delivering teleradiology services are already recognizable [25]. The Nighthawk model (named after the company that was first in the market) relocates fully licensed domestic radiologists to a country eight to 12 time zones ahead of the home country. Nighthawks pay their radiologist employees the prevailing domestic wage. This model has a number of advantages, including (1) compliance with existing licensure systems and (2) hospitals doing business with Nighthawks do not need to fear being sued for negligent hiring or supervising of their radiology staff. The chief disadvantages of Nighthawk services are that (1) relocating domestic radiologists overseas only perpetuates labor shortages in the home market and (2) the model is not a price-competitive alternative to traditional radiology.

The alternative to Nighthawk teleradiology is the Indian model (named after the country making the greatest use of this model). Indian providers hire unlicensed indigenous radiologists who are willing to work for one tenth the wages of radiologists in developed countries. Although hospitals in developed countries take on increased liability when they purchase teleradiology services from Indian teleradiologists, these hospitals can profit handsomely on the spread between domestic reimbursement for radiology services and the expense of the Indian teleradiologists. Thus, price-competitive Indian teleradiologists are more likely than Nighthawks to drive the expansion of the global market for teleradiology. Nor is it surprising that radiologists in developed countries are already lobbying for trade barriers to keep Indian teleradiology providers out of their market. The problem with such a business strategy is that trade barriers become ineffective with time [21].

This chapter examines macroeconomic and regulatory issues associated with trade in teleradiology [15]. Section 20.2 briefly discusses why the Indian teleradiologists have an absolute price advantage. However, trade in services is driven by comparative advantage and not absolute price advantage. After discussing the Ricadian and Heckscher–Ohlin (H-O) models for determining comparative advantage, we concluded that although India is unlikely to dominate trade in teleradiology, the market is still likely to expand in aggregate. Section 20.3 begins with an explanation of why medical licensure and trade barriers are unlikely to effectively regulate global trade in teleradiology. Then two novel suggestions on how trade in teleradiology might be effectively regulated are offered. We concluded that now is the time to open up international dialogue on how to regulate the Indian model for teleradiology.

20.2
Economic Issues

Getting into the global teleradiology market is not difficult. In addition to physician labor, one needs only access to a telecommunication package (computer, medical-grade software, and a virtual provider network) and a marketing method. The telecommunication package can be secured for less than US $150,000. This figure is easily affordable—although radiologists in developing countries may, depending on their business plan, have to pay more to finance the transaction. Thus, radiologists from developing countries who have the right marketing connections can enter the global market for teleradiology services almost as easily as radiologists from developed countries.

Once in the market, however, developing country radiologists have an important advantage: their physician labor costs are substantially less. This means that developing country teleradiologists can undercut the prices of their first-world competition. Indeed, India's market for exporting diagnostic testing, which is growing at the rate of 20% per year, earned US $864 million in 2005. Fear of the "India price" for teleradiology services has the American College of Radiology (ACR) already lobbying for market protection [4]. Yet the ACR could be overreacting to the threat of foreign competition because trade in teleradiology, like trade in any service, is determined by comparative advantage.

20.2.1
Ricardian Model

Whether a country has a comparative advantage depends on which economic model is used. With the Ricardian model, the country with the lowest opportunity costs has the comparative advantage. Opportunity costs, which are not necessarily all monetary, refer to what a country must give up in order to produce a service. When radiologists are employed in the export market, they are unavailable to provide their services to the domestic market. So, the opportunity costs of exporting teleradiology are those expenses associated with decreased access to radiology services in a domestic market [28].

Currently, in many developing countries, the opportunity costs associated with the exportation of teleradiology services are minimal. This is because many developing countries functionally deny health care to many of their citizens. For example, India with 1.1 billion people spends 5.1% of its gross domestic product (GDP) on health care [30]. This figure is a bit misleading because India only spends 0.9% of its GDP on health care for rural regions, where 70% of India's population lives. India's spending pattern helps explain the distributions of its medical facilities. India has only 22 "superspecialty hospitals" with telemedical capabilities that connect to only 78 remote locations [5]. As most of India's population has virtually no access to health care, India's opportunity costs for teleradiology are minimal because its citizenry is unlikely to notice any reduction in access to radiology services. A similar situation exists in China [20].

Yet, at a time when computers are being sold to the rural poor of developing nations [17], it seems likely that India's nonurban population will soon discover the quality of care they are missing. When Japan realized that its quality of health care lagged behind that of other industrialized counties, the Japanese began demanding Western-style health care [16]. But it is hard to imagine how India's (or any country's) economy can export telemedicine while providing Western-style health care to 16% of the world's population. As recently as in 1949, the disparate living conditions of the rural peasantry served as a driving force behind the Chinese revolution [9]. Indeed, even a causal reading of Fishman's book [9] demonstrates that opportunity costs arising from the denial of care to large segments of a society remain an important economic force.

Moreover, nothing ruins a country faster than a rapid influx of easy money [7]. If India should be successful in exporting significant volumes of teleradiology to the USA, money will flow into the country, resulting in rising domestic prices for radiology services. As only 10% of India's population has any form of health insurance coverage, rising radiology prices will mean that most patients in India will have to pay more out-of-pocket money for radiographic examinations [6]. In a country already skeptical of the "trickle-down" benefits from outsourcing, higher prices for radiology services are likely to stimulate social unrest [12].

20.2.2
H-O Model

Applying Ricardo's model to teleradiology has two limitations. First, Ricardo explicitly assumed that productivity was dependent solely on labor, whereas teleradiology production depends on both labor and labor's language skills [8]. Second, Ricardo implicitly assumed that productivity varied in different countries owing to access to technology, but in the global teleradiology market all providers will use virtually identical technology.

In contrast, the H-O model for international trade, which allows for multiple factors to impact productivity, is not encumbered by the Ricardian limitations. The H-O model predicts that a country, which produces services that consume factors it has in abundance, will have a comparative advantage. While a detailed discussion of H-O analysis for teleradiology is beyond the scope of this chapter, the impact of H-O theory on trade in teleradiology services can be observed by focusing on the impact of language. (Discussion of the language factor for teleradiology production was selected because no matter how accurate a radiographic interpretation be, if it miscommunicates clinical information, patients can be harmed. India is again used to illustrate the barriers that a developing country faces in the global teleradiology market.)

India and the USA each have about 800,000 physicians. India, however, has a population four times the size of that of the UASA, and only one third of India's physicians speak some English [15]. Thus, on a per capita basis, India has only 1/12th as many English-speaking physicians as the USA. For radiologists, the relative abundance of radiologists in the two countries is even more skewed: India has 5,500 radiologists compared with the 27,000 radiologists in the USA (a ratio of 1:50) [19]. If we forget about the fact that India exports teleradiology to the UK (and other English-speaking countries) and assume that all English-speaking Indian radiologists are fluent in English, even then, relative to the USA, India does not have an abundance of English-speaking radiologists. Indeed, Levy and Yu [19] have estimated that as few as 15 English-speaking radiologists comprise India's entire market for exporting teleradiology services to the USA.

So, while a few entrepreneurial Indian radiologists may do business with American hospitals, H-O analysis suggests that India does not have a comparative advantage over the USA in teleradiology. Significant exportation of teleradiology services from India to the USA is therefore not expected, nor is it likely that India's absolute price will determine the global market price.

20.2.3
Implications

This is not to say that the Indian model for teleradiology has no value. On the contrary, the Indian model may impact the American health-care market (1) indirectly through medical tourism, (2) in aggregate if widely adopted by other developing countries, and (3) by potentially stimulating a black market.

Broadly defined, medical tourism is the delivery of cost-effective private health care delivered in the context of a vacation [26]. This market, which primarily concerns surgical operations, is driven by economics. In essence, using a modification of the Indian model for teleradiology delivery, low-waged surgeons in the medical tourism countries can substantially undercut the prices of first-world surgeons. Based on the absolute price advantage for coronary artery bypass grafting (CABG) surgery in the medical tourism market, it is estimated that 30% of patients in need of elective CABG in the USA may be enticed to purchase this service abroad [27]. But purchasing an operation like a CABG in the medical tourism market results in lot of routine radiographic imaging being outsourced. So if large volumes of elective surgery move offshore, (1) the demand for radiologists in the USA is likely to fall and (2) the market for teleradiologists in developing countries is likely to grow, as they provide image interpretation for domestic surgeons in the medical tourism market.

In aggregate, the impact of trade in teleradiology may also negatively impact American radiologists. The English-speaking countries of the Southern Hemisphere (ESCSH)—Australia, New Zealand, and South Africa—may enter the global market. Today Australia's radiologists are primarily using the Nighthawk model, and New Zealand is importing teleradiology services from Indian providers. However, nothing prevents these countries from shifting their business model or trading policies. As radiologists in the ESCSH make substantially less money than American radiologists, the ESCSH could use the Indian model to export teleradiology to the USA. Like in India, radiologists in the ESCSH would have an absolute price advantage over American radiologists. But unlike in India, radiologists in the ESCSH would not have to face a language barrier. Conceivably, the lack of a language barrier and the price advantage could provide the ESCSH with a comparative advantage in teleradiology.

Finally, the Indian model for teleradiology is a paradigm for the creation of a black market. American hospitals face razor-thin profit margins, falling reimbursement, and increasing regulation, which erodes their ability to cross-subsidize patient care [3]. To cope with increasing financial instability, American hospitals will need to cut costs (amongst other things). Operating in such an environment, some hospitals are likely to take risks they otherwise would not. Indeed, it is not hard to imagine that a financially strained American hospital would elect to do business with Indian teleradiologists in order to cut costs. This raises an interesting question: How should countries protect their consumers from unlicensed physicians?

20.3
Legal Issues

Historically, licensure systems and trade barriers were the primary mechanisms by which countries protected their domestic markets from foreign and black market competition. These techniques work fairly well for trade in goods when enforced through gunboat diplomacy. Unfortunately for trade in services, including teleradiology, these methods are becoming increasingly ineffective in the global market: Licensure systems are difficult to enforce, and trade barriers are rapidly rendered obsolete by technology.

20.3.1
Licensure Technicalities

In general, for a country to enforce its licensure law on a foreign teleradiology provider, the disciplining country must demonstrate that (1) the foreign physicians receive proper notice (i.e., service of process), (2) the physician's home country must agree to extradite the teleradiologists, and (3) disciplining country must have personal jurisdiction. Legal technicalities at each of these levels create loopholes that allow unscrupulous foreign teleradiology providers to escape liability. First, there is the considerable procedural complexity of serving process in a foreign country. Unlike what is depicted by Hollywood, law enforcement agents from one country are not allowed to walk up to a defendant in another country and hand the defendant a summons and complaint. Rather, service of process on a foreign defendant must be conducted according to the dictates of an international treaty or the rules of the country where a defendant is located.

Once a summons has been served, a disciplining country must get the defendant's home country to agree to extradition. In general, a country rarely extradites its citizens unless the defendant is charged with a capital criminal offense. And because violations of medical licensure laws are rarely capital offenses, few countries extradite their physicians. Moreover, countries may refuse to extradite their teleradiologists because doing so would be contrary to the country's economic policies. For example, India's trade policy is to capture a greater share of the American health-care market [14]. So, in India any radiologist who exported millions of dollars of teleradiology services to the USA would be a patriot, and India, like all countries, rarely extradites its patriots.

Finally, prior to disciplining a foreign physician, a country's courts must have personal jurisdiction over the physician. Personal jurisdiction, in turn, arises when a defendant has had purposeful "minimal contacts" within a court's geographic jurisdiction. Again a detailed discussion on minimal contact analysis is beyond the scope of this chapter. However, as a general rule, minimal contacts are only created when a defendant *initiates* a transaction or uses property within a court's geographic jurisdiction. Just operating a Web site does not create minimal contacts [13]. Nor are minimal contracts necessarily created by an intermediary who introduced foreign teleradiologists to a hospital. The complexity of demonstrating minimal contract can be glimpsed in *Bradley vs Mayo Clinic*, a case where international concerns are minimized [1]. Although the Mayo Clinic's physicians actively managed the care of a patient in Kentucky, a Kentucky court ruled that it lacked personal jurisdiction over the Clinic. It seems likely that a Kentucky court would reach a similar conclusion if asked to hear a case involving a Bangalore teleradiologist who interpreted a radiograph of a Kentucky patient.

20.3.2
Trade Barriers

Alternatively, trade barriers might be used to protect the American radiology market. Any regulation that *unduly* increases transaction costs to a point where the purchase of services becomes cost-prohibitive is a trade barrier. Despite the current small size of the global market for teleradiology, the potential for price competition has the ACR lobbying for trade barriers in the form of onerous licensure requirements, demanding peer review, and mandating cost-prohibitive medical malpractice coverage [2]. In addition to restrictions on Medicare fund transfers, other novel trade barriers that might be employed to keep Indian teleradiologists out of the market include restrictions on Health Savings Account funds transfers and imposing security requirements on data-file transmission [11].

Economic history, however, teaches that trade barriers become less effective over time. Ultimately, the competition finds a way to neutralize a trade barrier. This is particularly true during the past 30 years, as technology has substantially reduced the life expectancy of trade barriers [10]. For example, within a month of China's demand that Google censor its searches, software to defeat Google's censor was available in the Chinese marketplace [29]. Such experiences suggest that ultimately the USA will not be able to protect its health-care market by erecting trade-communication barriers.

Technical erosion is not the only challenge to barriers designed to protect the American radiology market. Patient care advocates and insurers may lobby the

US Government for greater access for low-cost foreign teleradiology providers [32]. Importation of low-cost foreign teleradiology services would save patients and insurers money. Political pressure may also be brought to remove barriers to free trade in teleradiology by members of the World Trade Organization (WTO). The General Agreement on Trade in Services (GATS), which controls the WTO and covers medical services, calls for a country to remove trade barriers once a country makes a commitment to free trade in a particular service. At present, WTO trade negotiations have stalled over agriculture subsidies, and the USA has not made a meaningful commitment regarding its health-care sector. However, if negotiations at the WTO should begin again in earnest, developing countries may demand access to the American health-care market, the largest market in the world. So the ACR may lobby for trade barriers; if the USA is to continue to expand its capital markets overseas the quid pro quo may be the USA's commitment of its radiology sector to free trade.

20.3.3
Alternative Market Regulation

In short, something more than licensure systems and trade barriers will be needed to regulate the global teleradiology market. Alternatively, regulation of trade in teleradiology may be improved by using Internet architecture and/or market self-regulating methods.

For years, the Internet seemed to be the last bastion of anarchy. Early Internet protocols and related software were not capable of identifying who sent information. In the last 5–10 years, however, Internet users are no longer anonymous. Internet messages now include the sender's user name and IP address. With this information and "reverse look-up" software, any Internet transmission can be easily traced back to its origin. Lessig [18] has suggested that this maturation of the Internet could be used to credential the Internet user. Internet credentialing might be done by transmitting a password or by biometric technology (e.g., electronic thumbprint or retina scan), depending on the degree of security desired. Authentication/credentialing could even occur automatically by adding a new layer of protocol to the existing Internet architecture. Even if the Internet is not restructured, commercial credentialing software is now available to achieve this purpose [33].

These changes in Internet architecture could be used to regulate the global teleradiology market. Hospitals, for example, could be required to place credentialing filters in the firewalls of their servers. Assuming that a cost-effective method existed to identify an incoming radiology report from all other information flowing into a hospital, the identity of a radiology report sender could be verified by the modified firewall. The sender's identity could then be cross-referenced against a list of properly licensed radiologists. Reports from properly licensed radiologists would then be allowed to pass through the firewall to reach the treating physicians. If the sender was not an appropriately licensed radiologist, the report would be blocked at the firewall.

Authentication/credentialing software could represent an important improvement in quality control over the existing system of teleradiology reporting. Currently, it is all too easy for ghosting to occur in the global teleradiology market. On the other hand, architectural enforcement of licensure systems in cyberspace has the same limitation as a real-world licensure scheme: both are not self-enforcing. Certainly, authentication/credentialing software would detect more black market teleradiology transactions. However, without real-time regulation, teleradiologists and hospitals could still accept the risks of back-end litigation from black market transactions for the opportunity to make up-front profits.

Commodities exchange could be used as an alternative or a supplement to architectural methods for regulating the global market for teleradiology. Briefly, rather than allowing teleradiology transactions between hospitals and foreign radiologists to occur privately and in isolation, all teleradiology transactions would be funneled through a centralized exchange [24]. Radiologists would agree to deliver a certain volume of image interpretation to the exchange on a given day. Hospitals would then bid for these services much like commodities traders bid for agricultural, mineral, and financial services. Accordingly, teleradiology prices would be set by the market and not by a low bidder. Also, because of its central position in the market, the teleradiology exchange would credential providers, audit transactions, and certify the credit worthiness of purchasers. In essence, the exchange would act as a de facto global regulatory agency for teleradiology.

Implicit in this proposal is the need for a multilateral agreement to establish the exchange. Fortunately, because GATS covers teleradiology service, a new treaty would not need to be negotiated from scratch. GATS could be amended to create both the exchange and an enforcement mechanism to ensure that off-exchange transactions do not occur [22, 24]. In particular, signatories to GATS would agree that off-exchange teleradiology transactions (1) were per se criminal actions and (2) would subject providers to expeditious extradition proceeding. As criminal transactions, off-exchange teleradiology transactions would not entitle a provider to compensation. Moreover, hospitals caught purchasing off-exchange teleradiology services would waive their rights to use any country's judicial system to sue a telemedical provider after an adverse outcome. Collectively, these incentives are designed to make off-exchange teleradiology transactions prohibitively expensive for radiologists and hospitals.

Creation of a telemedical exchange would improve the transparency of international telemedical transactions at both the microeconomic and the macroeconomic levels. By driving all telemedical transactions through the exchange's servers, teleradiology would be more transparent and easier to regulate. At the macroscopic level, an exchange would provide a legitimate vehicle for foreign telemedical providers to meet the increasing demands of American patients for convenient and cost-effective routine medical care. By creating a legitimate and transparent forum for trade in teleradiology, the creation of a teleradiology commodities exchange would be a significant step toward minimizing a black market.

20.4
Conclusion

In the global market for teleradiology, providers from developing countries have an absolute price advantage because of their low-cost labor. The size of this market is subject to speculation and may currently be very small. Moreover, macroeconomic principles suggest that a single country may not be able to dominate the global teleradiology market. According to Ricardo's theory, rising opportunity costs may dissipate any comparative advantage of a developing country. The H-O theory suggests that language skills will further limit the comparative advantage of developing countries. On the other hand, the ESCSH may receive economic benefits from exporting teleradiology to the USA. So, in aggregate, trade in teleradiology may negatively impact the USAs' domestic radiology market.

Regardless of the ultimate size of the global market for teleradiology, more effective market-regulating mechanisms are needed. Traditional licensure systems are of limited use in the global market. Loopholes in services of process, extradition, and jurisdiction make medical licensure enforcement difficult at best. Moreover, as we progress in the twenty-first century, medical licensure systems are likely to find themselves at odds with the regulation of the WTO. Similarly, trade barriers are unlikely to protect a teleradiology market because of the rapidity of their technical obsolesce. Accordingly, now is the time to begin negotiations with other countries, perhaps under the auspices of the WTO, to regulate teleradiology by nontraditional methods. Modification of Internet architecture would help eliminate ghost interpretation of radiographic images, but the creation of a global teleradiology commodities exchange would improve market transparence while simultaneously creating an effective enforcement mechanism.

Summary

- In the global market for teleradiology, a developing country has an absolute price advantage.
- Opportunity costs and language skills will limit how much teleradiology a country can export.
- Better market regulation may be achieved by modification of the Internet's architecture or the commoditization of the market.

References

1. (1999) U.S. DIST. LEXIS 17505 (E.D. KY) Bradley v. Mayo Foundation, 1999 U.S. Dist. LEXIS 17505 (E.D. Ky. 1999)
2. Alexander AA (2007) American diagnostic teleradiology moves offshore: is the field riding the "Internet wave" into abyss? J Law Health 20:199–251
3. Altman SH, Shactman, Eilat E (2006) Could U.S. hospitals go the way of U.S. airlines? Health Affairs 25(1):11–21
4. American College of Radiology (2006) Revised statements on the interpretation of radiologic images outside the United States. http://www.acr.org/s_arc/doc.asp?CID=541&DID=24137. Accessed 28 April 2008
5. Bagchi S (2006) Telemedicine in rural India. PLoS Med 3(3):e82. doi: 10.1371/0030082
6. Bhatia P (2004) Health insurance in India. http://www.pitt.edu/~super1/lecture/lec19571/001.htm. Accessed 28 April 2008
7. Bonner W, Wiggins A (2006) Empire of debt. Wiley, Totowa
8. Bruzzi JF (2006) The words count-radiology and medical linguistics. N Engl J Med 354(7):665–667
9. Fishman TC (2005) China, Inc.: how the rise of the next superpower challenges America and the world. New York: Scribner
10. Friedman TL (1999) The Lexus and the olive tree. Farrar, Straus and Giroux, New York
11. Health savings accounts: missed opportunities. Medical Tourism Insights (2007). http://www.medicaltourismsinsight.com/articles/0702-hsa.htm. Accessed 28 April 2007
12. Hosalkar A (2007) As an Indian American I have to think ten times before investing a penny in India–India betrayed expatriate Indians on all accounts. India Dly. http://www.indiadaily.com/editorial.15086.asp. Accessed 28 April 2008
13. Hy Cite Corp. v. Badbusinessbureau.com, 297 F. Suppl 1154, 1160–4 (W.D. Wis. 2004)
14. India Representative to WHO (2004) Mode 1 services in health care. http://64.233.167.104/search?q=cache:WSVzDSlO_BoJ:www.whoindia.org/EIP/GATS/06-16.pdf+%22Mode+1+Services+in+Healthcare%22&hl=en&lr=lang_en. Accessed 16 Sep 2006
15. Konana P (2006) The healthcare tourism conundrum. Hindu. http://www.hinduonnet.com/2006/11/24/stories/2006112402361000.htm. Accessed 24 Jan 2007
16. Launders P (2007) Japan's 'cancer refugees' demand more options. Wall St J 11 January 2007, A1
17. (2007) Lenovo will sell computers to rural China. Kans City Star. http://www.kansascity.com/business/story/217807.html. Last Accessed 28 April 2008
18. Lessig L (2006) Code version 2.0. Basic Books, New York

19. Levy F, Yu K (2007) Offshoring radiology services to India. Massachusetts Institute of Technology. http://web.mit.edu/ipc/publications/pdf/06-005.pdf. Accessed 28 April 2008

20. McLean TR (2006) International law, telemedicine & health insurance: China as a case study. Am J Law Med 32(1):7–51

21. McLean TR (2006) The future of telemedicine & its Faustian reliance on regulatory trade barriers for protection. Health Matrix 16(2):443–509

22. McLean TR (2006) The legal and economic forces that will shape the international market for cybersurgery. Int J Med Robot 2(4):293–298

23. McLean TR (2007) Commoditization of the international teleradiology market. Journal of Health Services Research and Policy, 12:120–122

24. McLean TR (2007) Telemedicine and the commoditization of medical services. DePaul. J Health Care L. 135, 165

25. McLean TR, Richards EP (2006) Teleradiology: a case study of the economic and legal considerations in international trade in telemedicine. Health Affairs 25(5):1378–1385

26. (2005) Medical Tourism is becoming a common form of vacationing. Health Care Manage. http://www.expresshealthcaremgmt.com/20050315/medicaltourism02.shtml. Accessed 28 April 2008

27. Milstein A, Smith M (2007) Will the surgical world become flat? Health Affairs 26(1):137–141

28. Nagarajan SS (2006) International trade in healthcare services. Express Healthcare Manage. http://www.expresshealthcaremgmt.com/200611/analysis01.shtml. Accessed 28 April 2008

29. (2006) Outrunning China's web cop. Bus Week Online. http://www.businessweek.com/magazine/content/06_08/b3972061.htm. Accessed 28 April 2008

30. ProCOR (2006) Discussion policy. http://www.procor.org/discussion/displaymsg.asp?ref=2515&cate=ProCOR+Dialogue. Accessed 28 April 2008

31. Steinbrook R (2007) The age of telemedicine. N Engl J Med 357(1):5–7

32. Stokes B (2007) Protectionism and politics. U.S. Department of State's Bureau of International Information Programs. http://usinfo.state.gov/journals/ites/0107/ijee/stokes.htm. Accessed 28 April 2008

33. Michael V Copeland (2007) We don't need no stinkin' lawyers. Business 20 August 2007, pp 23–24

21

Teleradiology: An Audit

Sajeesh Kumar

Abstract Health-care providers are now looking at teleradiology as a model of improving, automating, and enhancing patient care. Available teleradiology technology still has considerable room for improvement. However, the challenge is why, where, and how to implement which technology and at what costs. A needs assessment is critical before implementing a teleradiology project.

21.1
Teleradiology Is Advancing

Teleradiology is a relatively young medical technology; consequently, further long-term study with regard to patient advantages, cost-effectiveness, and safety is required before the technology can be integrated into the mainstream health-care system. Teleradiology services are not going away, but the field is changing. As with many young industries, teleradiology seems to redefine itself on a fairly regular basis—changing to meet the demand of managing more and larger diagnostic images. The market is growing worldwide annually, owing, in large part, to the approval of procedures. In addition, given better acceptance in the general marketplace among radiologists, surgeons, hospitals, and patients, this growth will likely increase. It must be noted that the growth of imaging and telecommunication technologies will directly support and help the growth of teleradiology because these are, of course, an integral part of teleradiology.

21.2
Will Teleradiology Replace Traditional Methods?

Teleradiology promises to revolutionize health care and speed up the health-care process. Yet, the technology requires a great deal of further development. The coming of teleradiology does not mean that radiologists can abandon traditional methods. As well, the economics of teleradiology must be further analyzed. Institutions must ensure that the cost of teleradiology does not exceed the traditional expenses involved with radiology.

21.3
Issues Related to Teleradiology: A Brief Overview

Immediate or widespread implementation of teleradiology is hindered by many factors. The two biggest ones to be sorted out are the status of overseas reading of images and the evolving role of the virtual radiology department. Issues such as interpretation quality, reimbursement, and security are still in flux.

Issues related to teleradiology may also include lack of telecommunication infrastructure, affordability of programs, cost of the equipment, accuracy of the medical and nonmedical devices used, training of personnel involved, lack of guidelines and protocols, sustainability of the projects, regulations regarding sharing of information, privacy, and legal liability.

21.4
Changing Industry

While the location issue needs to be resolved, the nature of teleradiology services has greater long-term impact on the future of radiology practice. What will teleradiology practice look like in the coming years? To what extent and when might teleradiology replace on-site radiologists?

Teleradiology is driven by the relative shortage of radiologists and the rising number of images to be interpreted, not by the enabling technology. For the foreseeable future, getting all the images read will be the issue, not competition between teleradiology organizations and traditional groups.

The reality is that the local radiologist has much control of this situation. The local radiologist has the existing long-term community relationships and the ability to do procedures, on-site consultations, and conferences, as well as medical oversight in the radiology department. Most local radiology groups have exclusive contracts with the hospitals. Radiology groups choose to do business with teleradiology companies with reputations that they can trust. The biggest risk that a local radiology group can take is to continue in a seriously understaffed situation. By partnering with a trusted teleradiology provider, they should find out that their local hospital contract is more secure than it ever has been. Anything that improves service in the local practice will, in the form of better staffing levels, make it much harder for an outsider to compete.

If hospitals and groups have an on-site option, they are going to take it. Even sites with radiology groups in place are looking for someone to handle the overflow. A radiology group might read for five or six hospitals and use teleradiology to shift work among its members. It may also contract with a teleradiology company to handle overflow. Expansion may come in daytime teleradiology because that is simply when most studies are being done. Of course, physicians' turnaround expectations are getting shorter, not longer.

21.5
Technical Challenge

One technical challenge to teleradiology's daytime expansion is the availability of patients' prior examination and other data. Efficiently linking teleradiology providers to patients' prior data is an important step toward replicating the service of in-house radiology through teleradiology. Of course, it requires that the originating hospitals have IT systems in place to provide the information. Implementing this access could be the next quantum step in teleradiology development.

21.6
Money Matters

Meeting the demand is a major teleradiology driver, along with economic motivation. A group already large enough to staff and share off-hour calls may show an economic benefit. Given imaging demand, radiologist lifestyle, and economic factors, teleradiology services are not going away, but the field is rapidly changing. Besides quality radiologists, a track record of adaptability might be that the trait facilities and groups need to focus on when they consider implementing teleradiology technology.

Financial planning for teleradiology should include the costs of telecommunication and information technology infrastructure and medical devices, as well as costs such as personnel training, monthly network access fees, maintenance, telephone bills, and other operational expenses.

Once the objectives of a program have been identified, technology support personnel should be consulted, to clarify technical equipment specifications and facility requirements. Protocols and guidelines must be developed, which will provide clear direction on how to utilize teleradiology most effectively. The training of operators is especially critical in teleradiology. The reliability of a program is also related to the experience with teleradiology technology and the awareness of its limitations.

Many nations do not have explicit policies to pay for teleradiology services. A major teleradiology payment policy is crucial. Meanwhile, several telemedicine services are being integrated into regular health-care systems in the USA and the Scandinavian countries with reimbursement/payment options. Studies should be conducted to implement, monitor, evaluate, and refine the teleradiology payment process. Additionally, it should be noted that teleradiology licensure and indemnity laws might also need to be formulated. This issue, however, remains a cloudy region for health-care strategists and has implications for radiologists and remote practitioners who practice across state or country lines.

It is observed that successful teleradiology programs are often the product of careful planning, sound management, dedicated professionals and support staff, and a commitment to appropriate funding to support capital purchases and ongoing operations. It reflects a commitment to teamwork to link technical and operational complexities into a fully integrated and efficiently functioning program. Teleradiology service providers, health insurance agencies, and all institutions concerned could convene to lead a workable model for teleradiology service improvements. The professional communities could bring out teleradiology service guidelines, which would pave the way for consensus on several difficult issues, including technical and service standardization for teleradiology.

21.7
Conclusion

Health-care providers are now looking at teleradiology as a model of improving, automating, and enhancing patient care. This book elaborates on many aspects of teleradiology. The authors have shown teleradiology to be practical, safe, and effective. Success often relates to the efficiency and effectiveness of the transfer of information and translates to improved or enhanced patient care, compared with traditional methods.

Available teleradiology technology still has considerable room for improvement. However, the challenge is why, where, and how to implement which technology and at what costs. Asking the right questions will drive the technologies. A needs assessment is critical before implementing a teleradiology project. Teleradiology, as delineated in these pages, may appear novel but is rapidly coming into common and mundane usage through multiple applications. Time alone will tell whether teleradiology (to paraphrase Neil Armstrong) is "one small step for information and communication technology but one giant leap for radiology." However, from the pages of this first-ever book on teleradiology, the future promises to be exciting. Optimistically, the journey toward improved patient care will be well worth the wait for those benefiting from these technologies.

Bibliography

1. Jakobsen KR (2002) Space-age medicine, stone-age government: how Medicare reimbursement of telemedicine services is depriving the elderly of quality medical treatment. Health Care Law 274:9–37
2. Knaub J (2007) Teleradiology transforming. Radiol Today 6(4):22

Glossary

ActiveX ActiveX is a Microsoft technology used for developing reusable object oriented software components.

ActiveX data object Can be used to access databases from your Web pages.

Advanced encryption standard An encryption standard now used by the US Government, which replaced the older standard data encryption standard. It is now commonly featured in many wireless products.

Angiogram An X-ray is used to visualize the opening of a blood vessel. Typically contrast is injected intravenously in order to highlight the blood flow.

Asynchronous transfer mode A telecommunications protocol that encodes data traffic into small fixed-sized cells.

Augmented reality A field of computer research that deals with the combination of real-world and computer-generated data.

802.11b Standard for wireless local-area networks (WLANs), also often called Wi-Fi and is part of the 802.11 series of WLAN standards from the Institute of Electrical and Electronics Engineers (IEEE).

Bluetooth A short-range wireless connection between electric devices, most commonly mobile phones and other devices, including computers.

Borland Borland Software Corporation is a software company.

bps Bits per second: speed at which the transfer of data is measured over an Internet connection.

Bps   Bytes per second: another measure of transfer speed over an Internet connection. (1 byte 8 bits).

Cathode ray tube   A display monitor that works by scanning an electron beam across the back of the screen, lighting up phosphor on the inside of the glass tube, thereby illuminating portions of the screen.

COM+   An extension of component object model, Microsoft's strategic building-block approach for developing application programs.

Computed radiography   A digital imaging system that uses a storage phosphor plate as the image detector. A laser beam scans the latent image on the storage plate to yield a digital image.

Computed tomography   An imaging method where digital processing is used to generate a 3D image from a large series of 2D X-ray images taken around a single axis of rotation.
     A series of two-dimensional X-rays, ideal when looking at a hemorrhage, skeletal structure, or ionic salts (stones).

Computer cluster   A group of tightly coupled computers that work together closely so that in many respects they can be viewed as though they are a single computer.

Cross-enterprise document sharing for images (XDS-I) integration profile   In order to solve the integration problems of the development of an electronic health-care record system in the inability to share and exchange patient records among various hospitals and health-care providers, Integrating Healthcare Enterprise (IHE) has defined an integration profile called cross-enterprise document sharing (XDS) to regulate the sharing of data contained in medical records. The XDS for imaging (XDS-I) integration profile, depending on the IHE XDS integration profile, extends and specializes XDS to support imaging "documents," specifically including sets of digital imaging and communication in medicine (DICOM) instances (including images, evidence documents, presentation states, and diagnostic imaging reports provided in a ready-for-display format).

Data authenticity   Refers to validating the source of a message and ensuring that it was transmitted by a properly identified sender.

Data integrity   Refers to the assurance that the data were not modified accidentally or deliberately in transit, by replacement, insertion, or deletion.

Data privacy   Refers to denying access to information by unauthorized individuals.

Digital imaging and communication in medicine   An international organization of users and vendors for standardization in medical imaging.

A standard for interconnection of medical digital imaging devices. It was developed by the American College of Radiology and the National Electrical Manufacturers Association. It consists of a standard image file format and a standard communications protocol.

A standard that was developed by the American College of Radiology and the National Electrical Manufacturers Association in 1993 to promote communication of digital image information, regardless of device manufacturer; to facilitate the development and expansion of picture archiving and communication systems, which can also interface with other systems; and to allow the creation of diagnostic information databases, which can be interrogated by a wide variety of devices distributed geographically.

DICOM communication with IPSec-based security   The security features of DICOM image communication services over TCP/IPv4 or TCP/IPv6 are provided by using IPSec.

DICOM image communication with SSL/TLS-based security   The security features of DICOM image communication services over TCP/IPv4 or TCP/IPv6 are provided by using the SSL/TLS protocol.

DICOM image secure communication   The transfer of DICOM images through a public network with security measures to ensure the privacy, authenticity, and integrity of the data.

DICOM upper-layer protocols with TCP/IPv4   DICOM uses the OSI upper-layer service to separate the exchange of DICOM messages or objects at the application layer from the communication support provided by the lower layers. This OSI upper-layer service boundary allows peer application entities to establish associations, transfer messages, and terminate associations. The DICOM upper-layer protocol with TCP/IPv4 is the upper-layer protocol augmenting TCP/IPv4 that is adopted by DICOM communication applications to implement DICOM communication services to transfer or deliver DICOM messages or image objects between equipments or devices.

DICOM upper layer with TCP/IPv6   The DICOM upper-layer protocol with TCP/IPv6 is the upper-layer protocol augmenting TCP/IPv6 that is adopted by DICOM communication applications to implement DICOM communication services to transfer or deliver DICOM messages or image objects between equipments or devices.

Digital radiography A digital imaging system that captures image data in digital format.

eHealth The application of information and communications technologies across the whole range of functions that affect the health sector, from the physician to the hospital manager, via nurses, data-processing specialists, social security administrators and—of course—the patient (European Union definition).

Electronic health-care record (EHR) A longitudinal electronic record of patient health information generated by one or more encounters in any care delivery setting. Included in this information are patient demographics, progress notes, problems, medications, vital signs, past medical history, immunizations, laboratory data, and radiology reports. The EHR automates and streamlines the clinician's workflow. The EHR has the ability to generate a complete record of a clinical patient encounter, as well as supporting other care-related activities directly or indirectly via an interface, including evidence-based decision support, quality management, and outcomes reporting.

Extensible authentication protocol An authentication framework used commonly in wireless networks, of which the Wi-Fi protected access (WPA) and WPA2 are adopted subtypes.

Haptic Force, velocity, grasp, and even temperature feeling.

Health Insurance Portability and Accountability Act US legislation that places strict requirements on security and privacy of health-care data of patients.

Hypertext transfer protocol (HTTP) An application-level protocol for distributed, collaborative, hypermedia information systems, which goes over TCP/IP connections and uses request/response operation models to transfer data. A client sends a request to the server in the form of a request method, URI, and protocol version, followed by a MIME-like message containing request modifiers, client information, and possible body content over a connection with a server. The server responds with a status line, including the message's protocol version and a success or error code, followed by a MIME-like message containing server information, entity meta-information, and possible entity body content.

Hypertext transfer protocol over secure socket layer (HTTPS)   A Web protocol originally developed by Netscape (now a subsidiary of America Online). It can encrypt and decrypt user page requests as well as the pages that are returned by the web server. HTTPS is really just the use of secure socket layer as a sublayer under its regular HTTP application layer. It uses a certificate and a public key to encrypt data to be transferred over the Internet.

ICD-10   The International Statistical Classification of Diseases and Related Health Problems — 10th revision (ICD-10) is a coding of diseases and signs, symptoms, abnormal findings, complaints, social circumstances, and external causes of injury or diseases, as classified by the World Health Organization.

Image communication modes in teleradiology   Image delivery in teleradiology operates in either "push" or "pull" modes. In push mode, the image data are sent to the expert site or expert center from the requester site directly using the point-to-point (simple and complicated teleradiology) and the many-to-point (expert-model teleradiology) models. In the push model, data transmission can be completed using the DICOM storage (C-Store) communication service. In pull mode, the requester first puts the image data in somewhere, notifying the expert that the image data are available; then, the expert first finds the data and retrieve them. If the communication protocol of the pull mode uses DICOM, there will be at least two DICOM communication services: the DICOM storage service (C-Store SCU/SCP) and the DICOM query/retrieval service.

Integrating Healthcare Enterprise (IHE)   A multiyear initiative that creates the framework for passing vital health information seamlessly—from application to application, system to system, and setting to setting—across the entire health-care enterprise. Under the leadership of HIMSS and the Radiological Society of North America, IHE began in November 1998 as a collaborative effort to improve the way computer systems in health care share critical information. IHE includes medical specialists and other care providers, administrators, standards organizations, IT professionals, and vendors. In 2003, the American College of Cardiology joined the initiative as a sponsor, in order to advance cross-vendor integration for cardiovascular medicine. IHE does not create new standards but rather drives the adoption of standards to address specific clinical needs. IHE integration profiles specify precisely how standards are to be used to address these needs, eliminating ambiguities, reducing configuration and interfacing costs, and ensuring a higher level of practical interoperability.

Internet protocols   Indicates the communication protocols used by the current Internet to transmit information. The most commonly used protocols usually include TCP/IPv4, TCP/IPv6, HTTP, HTTPS, small object access protocol (SOAP), etc.

Internet protocol security (IPSec)   A member of the IPv6 family. It provides security to the IP and the upper-layer protocols. IPSec is composed of two protocols: authentication header (AH) protocol and encapsulating security payload (ESP) protocol. AH is used to ensure the authentication and integrity of message, while ESP is used to ensure confidentiality. The AH protocol uses hash message authentication codes to protect integrity. Many algorithms can be used in AH, such as secure hash algorithm, Message Digest-5, etc. The ESP protocol uses the standard symmetric encryption algorithms to protect confidentiality, such as triple data encryption standard, advanced encryption standard, 448-bit Blowfish encryption algorithm, etc.

Internet protocol version 6 (IPv6)   A new version of IP designed to be an evolutionary step of IPv4. IPv6 is designed to run well on high-performance networks (e.g., gigabit Ethernet, OC-12, ATM, etc.) and at the same time still be efficient for low-bandwidth networks (e.g., wireless). In addition, it provides a platform for higher-speed Internet functionality, which will be required in the near future. IPv6 was designed to solve many of the problems of the current version of IPv4 with regard to address depletion, security, autoconfiguration, extensibility, and others. IPv6 includes many associated protocols such as IPSec, ICMPv6, etc. IPv6 has some special features as follows: (1) larger address space; (2) aggregation-based address hierarchy and efficient backbone routing; (3) efficient and extensible IP datagram such as no fragmentation by routers, 64-bit field alignment, and simpler basic header; (4) autoconfiguration; (5) security; and (6) IP renumbering as part of the protocol.

Java applet   An applet delivered in the form of Java bytecode. Applets are used to provide interactive features to Web applications that cannot be provided by hypertext markup language (HTML).

Java beans   Classes written in the Java programming language conforming to a particular convention. They are used to encapsulate many objects into a single object (the bean) so that the bean can be passed around rather than the individual objects.

Java servlet   The Java servlet API allows a software developer to add dynamic content to a Web server using the Java platform. The content generated is commonly HTML but may be other data such as XML.

Joint Photographic Experts Group   JPEG. A digital image file format designed for maximal image compression.

Joint Photographic Experts Group format   Commonly used algorithm to compress photographic images with a mild loss in image quality.

kbps   Kilobits per second (1,000 bits = 1 kbps).

Liquid crystal display   A display monitor that uses two pieces of polarizing material with a liquid crystal solution in-between. An electric current passes through the liquid, making the crystals align so that light can pass.

Lightweight extensible authentication protocol   Proprietary WLAN authentication methoddeveloped by Cisco Systems, which among other things uses dynamic wired equivalent privacy keys.

Magnetic resonance imaging   Noninvasive imaging with no radiation exposure; typically has better resolution on living tissue than computed tomography.
  A noninvasive, nonionizing imaging technique based on magnetic fields of hydrogen atoms in the body.

Mbps   Megabits per second (1,000,000 bits = 1 Mbps).

Media access control division multiplexing   A unique identifier found on all network interface cards. It is possible to change the address on most hardware.

Multipurpose Internet   Internet standard that extends the format of **mail extension** e-mail to support.

.NET   The Microsoft .NET framework is a software component that can be added to or is included with the Microsoft Windows operating system. It provides a large body of precoded solutions to common program requirements and manages the execution of programs written specifically for the framework.

Orthogonal frequency   An algorithm to transmit signals commonly used in wireless networks.

Personal digital assistant   Handheld computers that have evolved into powerful computers capable of accessing large memory files and high-speed wireless networks.

A hand-held organizer that now typically has phone, Internet, and camera capabilities.

PHP hypertext preprocessor   A server-side HTML-embedded scripting language that provides Web developers with a full suite of tools for building dynamic websites.

Picture archiving and communication system   Computers or networks dedicated to the storage, retrieval, distribution, and presentation of images.

A networked medical imaging information communication and management system. It consists of many components such as image acquisition gateway, communication networks, image database and archiving devices or a storage subsystem, image processing, and display workstations. PACS can be a small local network system or can be enterprise widely connected and used in multiple hospitals. It provides a network environment and platform to allow radiology departments to realize filmless and cost-effective digital imaging diagnosis and enables the radiologists remotely to provide high quality of imaging diagnostic service in teleradiology.

A network of acquisition devices, computers, displays, and network equipment to acquire, store, transmit, and display digital medical images.

Pretty good privacy   A computer program that provides cryptographic privacy and authentication.

Public key infrastructure   An arrangement that binds public keys with respective user identities by means of a certificate authority.

Portable Network Graphics   A bitmapped image format that employs lossless data compression.

Protected extensible authentication protocol   A method to securely transmit authentication information; however, it is not an encryption protocol and only authenticates a client trying to gain access to a network.

Receiver operating characteristic   An analysis technique used to assess the diagnostic performance of radiologists.

Renal   Pertaining to kidneys.

Renal colic   A type of pain commonly caused by kidney stones in the kidney itself or also the bladder.

Secure file transfer protocol   A network protocol designed by the IETF to provide secure file transfer and manipulation facilities over the secure shell protocol.

Secure shell   A network protocol that allows data to be exchanged over a secure channel between two computers.

Secure socket layer/transfer-layer security (SSL/TLS)   The SSL was originally developed by Net-scape Communications to allow secured access of a browser to a Web server. SSL has become the accepted standard for Web security. It provides a secure communication channel between the client and the server by allowing mutual authentication, which uses digital signatures for integrity and encryption for privacy. The protocol was designed to support multiple choices of specific algorithms used for cryptography, digests, and signatures. The SSL protocol uses both public-key and symmetric-key encryptions. Symmetric-key encryption is much faster than public-key encryption, but public-key encryption provides better authentication techniques. SSL consists of two protocols: the handshake and the SSL record protocols. The handshake protocol defines how the peer entities exchange associated information, such as SSL version and ciphers, and authenticates certificates. The SSL record protocol defines the format of the SSL record or message, in which all of the SSL-associated messages or application data should be transferred. The SSL connection is executed in two phases: the first is handshake and the second is data transfer. SSL 3.0 is the basis for the TLS protocol, which is still being developed by the Internet Engineering Task Force.

Service class provider (SCP)   The role played by a DICOM application entity (DICOM message service element service user), which performs operations and invokes notifications on a specific association.

Service class user (SCU)   The role played by a DICOM application entity (DICOM message service element service user), which invokes operations and performs notifications on a specific association.

Simple mail transfer protocol   The de facto standard for e-mail transmissions across the Internet.
    Text-based protocol that allows a text message to be sent via e-mail.

Spyware   Computer software that is often installed on a personal computer without the knowledge of the user and that can take control of the computer.

Tagged Image File Format   A file format for storing images.

Tele-immersion   The integration of audio and video conferencing with collaborative virtual reality in the context of data-mining and significant computation.

Telemedicine   The investigation, monitoring, and management of patients and staff using systems that allow ready access to expert advice and patient information, no matter where the patient or relevant information is located (European Union definition).

Teleradiology   The electronic transmission of radiological patient images, such as X-rays, CT images, and MRI images, from one location to another for the purposes of interpretation and/or consultation (American College of Radiology definition).

Transmission control protocol/Internet protocol version 4 (TCP/IPv4)   TCP and IP were developed by a Department of Defense research project to connect a number different networks designed by different vendors into a network of networks (the "Internet"). IP is responsible for moving a packet of data from node to node, and TCP is responsible for verifying the correct delivery of data from client to server. Most network applications and protocols (client/server, Web, HTTP, DICOM, etc.) used in the Internet or an intranet are developed on the basis of TCP/IP, which is partitioned into three layers according to the International Standards Organization open systems interconnection definition, i.e., the application layer, the transport layer, and the IP layer. IPv4 is now nearly 20 years old and has been remarkably resilient in spite of its age; it forwards each packet based on a 4-byte destination address, but it is beginning to have the following problems: (1) address shortage, (2) security is not integrated and IPSec is an add-on, (3) problems of multicasting, (4) complicated header, (5) fragmentation/retransmission problems, (6) poor quality of service, (7) inability to handle large frames, and (8) limited autoconfiguration support (needed by dynamic host configuration protocol).

Ultrasound   High-frequency sound waves used to image soft tissues such as tendons, muscles, and organs.

Virtual private network   A communication network tunneled through another network and dedicated for a specific network.

Virtual reality   A technology that allows a user to interact with a computer-simulated environment, be it a real or an imagined one.

VisiBroker   Borland VisiBroker is the most widely deployed common object request broker architecture object request broker infrastructure product on the market.

Volume rendering   A technique used to display a 2D projection of a 3D discretely sampled data set.

Web access DICOM persistent object (WADO)   The DICOM standard specifies a Web-based service called WADO for accessing and presenting DICOM persistent objects (e.g., images and medical imaging reports). WADO is intended for distribution of results and images to health-care professionals. It provides a simple mechanism for accessing a DICOM persistent object from HTML pages or XML documents, using HTTP/HTTPS and DICOM unique identifiers. Data may be retrieved either in a presentation-ready form as specified by the requester (e.g., Joint Photographic Experts Group format or Graphics Interchange Format) or in a DICOM native format.

Wi-Fi   Wireless technology brand owned by the Wi-Fi Alliance intended to improve the interoperability of WLAN products, based on the IEEE 802.11 standards.

Wi-Fi protected access   A newer wireless encryption in response to the known weakness of wired equivalent privacy.

Windows NT   A family of operating systems produced by Microsoft.

Wired equivalent privacy   Wireless standard that allows encryption; however, it is considered insecure and is no longer recommended for use.

Subject Index

Printing: Krips bv, Meppel, The Netherlands
Binding: Stürtz, Würzburg, Germany